The Dysarthrias:

Physiology, Acoustics, Perception, Management

The Dysarthrias:

Physiology, Acoustics, Perception, Management

Edited by

Malcolm R. McNeil, PhD
University of Wisconsin
Madison, Wisconsin

John C. Rosenbek, PhD
VA Medical Center
Madison, Wisconsin

Arnold E. Aronson, PhD
The Mayo Clinic
Rochester, Minnesota

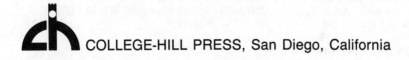 COLLEGE-HILL PRESS, San Diego, California

College-Hill Press
4284 41st Street
San Diego, California 92105

Library of Congress Cataloging in Publication Data

Main entry under title:

The Dysarthrias.

   Includes bibliographies and indexes.
   1. Articulation disorders. I. McNeil, Malcolm Ray. II. Rosenbek, John C.
III. Aronson, Arnold Elvin. [DNLM: 1. Speech disorders. WL 340 D9975]
RC424.7.D95   1984   616.85'5   83-14394

ISBN 0-933014-03-1

Contents

Contributors

James H. Abbs, PhD
Department of Communicative
  Disorders
Speech Motor Control Laboratories
University of Wisconsin
Madison, WI 53706

Arnold E. Aronson, PhD
Mayo Clinic
Rochester, MN 55901

James L. Aten, PhD
Veterans Administration
  Medical Center
5901 East Seventh Street
Long Beach, CA 90822

Celia J. Bassich, MA
Communicative Disorders Program
National Institute of Neurological &
  Communicative Disorders & Stroke
7550 Wisconsin Avenue, Room 1C-13
Bethesda, MD 20205

David R. Beukelman, PhD
Department of Rehabilitation
  Medicine, RJ-30
University of Washington
Seattle, WA 98195

Joe R. Brown, MD
1784 Alta Vista
Vista, CA 92083

Ray Gutierrez, CDT
Veterans Administration
  Medical Center
5901 East Seventh Street
Long Beach, CA 90822

Thomas J. Hixon, PhD
Department of Speech & Hearing
  Sciences
University of Arizona
Tucson, AZ 85721

Chauncey J. Hunker, MS
Speech Motor Control Laboratories
517 Waisman Center
1500 Highland Avenue
University of Wisconsin
Madison, WI 53706

Craig Linebaugh, PhD
Speech & Hearing Center
George Washington University
2201 G. Street NW
Washington, DC 20052

Christy Ludlow, PhD
NIH, NINCDS-CDP
7550 Wisconsin Avenue, Room 1C-12
Bethesda, MD 20205

Alonzo McDonald, DDS
Prosthetics Section
Veterans Administration
  Medical Center
5901 East Seventh Street
Long Beach, CA 90822

Malcolm R. McNeil, PhD
Department of Communicative
  Disorders
Speech Motor Control Laboratories
University of Wisconsin
Madison, WI 53706

Fred D. Minifie, PhD
Speech & Hearing Sciences
  Department, JG-15
University of Washington
Seattle, WA 98195

Ronald Netsell, PhD
Boys Town Institute for
  Communication Disorders in
  Children
555 N. 30th Street
Omaha, NE 68131

Anne H. B. Putnam, PhD
Department of Speech & Hearing
  Sciences
University of Arizona
Tuscon, AZ 85721

John C. Rosenbek, PhD
Audiology & Speech Pathology
Veterans Administration
2500 Overlook Terrace
Madison, WI 53705

Rick Rubow, PhD
Speech Motor Control Laboratories
R533 Waisman Center
1500 Highland Avenue
University of Wisconsin
Madison, WI 53706

Shimon Sapir, PhD
Department of Neurology
Mayo Clinic
Rochester, MN 59505

Marianne Simpson, MA
Speech Pathologist
Long Beach VA Medical Center

Gary Weismer, PhD
Speech Motor Control Laboratories
567 Waisman Center
1500 Highland Avenue
University of Wisconsin
Madison, WI 53706

Victoria E. Wolfe, MA
St. Anthony Hospital
Columbus, OH 43203

Kathryn M. Yorkston, PhD
Department of Rehabilitation
  Medicine, RJ-30
University of Washington
Seattle, WA 98195

Dedication

This book and companion text on apraxia of speech have grown from two perceived needs. The first is a need to provide a state of science review of the nature, assessment, and treatment of the dysarthrias and of apraxia of speech, along with the most prominent current research by the leading researchers in the field. This need has been addressed by providing a major review and projective essay preceding the original data-based contributions for the motor speech disorders.

The second, and equally important need grew from a desire to honor the time-unlimited contributions to motor speech disorders made by Dr. Frederic L. Darley on his formal retirement. His colleagues and his pre- and postdoctoral fellows at the Mayo Clinic initiated this tribute. In order to provide recognition of his profound impact on the field of motor speech disorders, on dysarthric and apraxic persons, and on all of us, this book is dedicated to him. Its scope reflects neither the trails traveled nor the passages opened by Dr. Darley. However, this book does reflect the fervor, diversity of approaches, and the intellectual honesty needed to address motor speech disorders. This fervor, diversity, and honesty he champions.

Malcolm R. McNeil
John C. Rosenbek
Arnold E. Aronson

Acknowledgments

We wish to acknowledge Debra Shimon, Brenda Kleinheinz, Kathy Lindgren, and Marilyn Parnell for their editorial and secretarial support. This work was in part supported by Grants NS 18797-01 and NS 13274-071 from the National Institute of Neurological and Communicative Disorders and Stroke.

Preface

Abnormalities of motor speech have long been used as clues to the type of neurologic dysfunction and as an aid to neurologic diagnosis. However, the judgments as to the type of abnormality were often based on an overall impression of abnormality described as dysarthric speech, or slurred speech. Other judgments selected abnormalities, such as scanning speech or festinating speech, considered to be specific for certain neurologic syndromes. On occasion, acoustic imagery has been evoked by phrases such as "hot potato speech." Prior to 1969 there were few organized studies of the specific deviations of speech in various motor system disorders. At that time Darley and colleagues identified, defined, and rated the deviant sounds encountered in dysarthrias of varied types. Subsequently, the acoustic characteristics of apraxia of speech were defined. It was concluded that the observed abnormalities of motor speech were determined by the part of the motor system that was impaired and the resultant specific neuromuscular defect (weakness, slowness, hypertonus, etc.). These abnormalities of motor speech should be verifiable by measurements of physiologic and neural functioning.

This book and the companion volume on apraxia of speech are an outgrowth and extention of those stated principles. This text opens with an overview of the dysarthrias, providing background information and furnishing a perspective. Following contributions are devoted to specifics, with an emphasis on information derived from measurements of acoustic, physiologic, or neuromuscular dysfunction in dysarthia and of acoustic, linguistic, or anatomic alterations in apraxia of speech. The final contributions in each section are devoted to treatment.

Joe R. Brown, MD
Vista, CA

1

A Neurobiologic View of the Dysarthrias

Ronald Netsell

PROLOGUE

A Definition of Dysarthria

This chapter emphasizes a neurobiologic view of individuals whose speech is considered to be dysarthric. Dysarthria is defined here as a *speech* disorder resulting from damage to *neural mechanisms* that *regulate* speech movements. The presence of "speech" in this definition is to distinguish dysarthria from language disorders (aphasias) or more broadly based cognitive disorders. The presence of "regulate" in the definition is to distinguish dysarthria from apraxia of speech, where the latter results from damage to neural mechanisms responsible for selecting, sequencing, and (perhaps) constructing the spatial-temporal goals of a given speech act.

A Neurobiologic View

In this chapter a neurobiologic view is developed that emphasizes evolutionary and biologic determinants of speech and its neurologic disorders. Optimal treatment of an individual with dysarthria represents the best fitting of available treatment procedures to our best *understanding* of the determinants of that individual's speech patterns. In seeking that understanding, a neurobiologic approach emphasizes the "interactionist model" of physiologic and external environmental variables (after Wolff, 1981).

> The "interactionist model" offers a viable alternative to either of the extreme for-
> mulations, because it can integrate data on both physiological (genetic, hormonal,
> neurological) and experiential determinants without a commitment to either factor
> as a sufficient cause...Physiologic processes prepare the organism to respond ap-
> propriately to environmental events that will promote its psychological and
> physiological development. Experience has potent physiological and structure ef-
> fects, as well as behavioral consequences. Therefore, the causal chain is as likely to
> proceed from experience to physiology and structure formation as from structure to
> behavior. (Wolff, 1981, p. 1)

The neurobiologic view presented here is that the current status of the human nervous system can best be understood against the background of (1) its evolution, including that of nonhuman primates (i.e., phylogeny), (2) the development of the individual's nervous system, as influenced by its phylogeny and interactions with its environment (i.e., ontogeny); and (3) the "survival value" of the behaviors of interest (in particular, the vocal expressions of emotion and thought).[1]

An Underlying Premise

The premise underlying the search for a better understanding of the dysarthrias is that this knowledge will benefit individuals with the prob-lem, as well as those who may suffer brain injury in the future. Whereas even 20 to 25 years ago there was little evidence that treatment could be a major influence in recovery from brain injury, current thinking and data reflect a considerable optimism (c.f., Bach-y-Rita, 1980; Finger & Stein, 1982). Another benefit of studying speech and neurologic conditions from a neurobiologic perspective should be an increase in our under-standing of the origins, extant behaviors, and future behaviors of human communication (in particular) and the hominid (in general). Two articles illustrate the above statements. Brodal (1973), a neuroanatomist, provid-ed insightful neurophysiologic hypotheses about the differential effects of spontaneous recovery and various therapies, based on self-observations following a stroke. Pribram (1982), in developing thoughts for a "neurobiologic theory of music," draws striking parallels to human language.

A Review of Reviews

Given some obvious limitations (including page allocation and the opi-nions of the author), this chapter necessarily represents a "review of reviews" in that many of the references cited are summaries of large bodies of information. As with any review, this one is selective and oversights in referencing as well as inaccuracies in interpretation are inevitable. To those who will feel slighted or misunderstood, I sympathize in advance.

The plan for this chapter is to (1) provide an historical perspective for the emergence of dysarthria as a topic for interdisciplinary study, (2) summarize more recent advances in understanding the nervous system, speech motor control, and neuropathophysiology, and (3) relate these issues to the treatment of dysarthria.

HISTORICAL DEVELOPMENTS

A neurobiologic view of the dysarthrias has traceable roots to individuals and groups who emphasized speech physiology, its evolutionary development, or both. This historical perspective pertains basically to those developments in the 20th century and in the United States. What seems clear is that parallel approaches were being developed in the US and USSR, and recent translations of Luria (1970, 1981) reveal the strong influence of the "interactionist model" in the Russians' view of human communication and its disorders. Indeed, by the definitions given above, the work of Pavlov, Bechterew, Schenkov, Anohkin, Bernstein, and Vygotsky was embodied by Luria in a truly neurobiologic sense. Luria emphasized a "functional systems" analysis of cognition/language/speech disorders, planning in his last years to move from cortical to subcortical influences, anticipating or paralleling, as always, the directions and development of other researchers.

1900–1950

The start of this period (1900-1950) seems most clearly marked to me by the dissertation of John Muyskens (1925) at the University of Michigan titled *The Hypha*. The hypha was regarded as a "physiological syllable" and represents a clear forerunner of the continuing search for "basic units" of speech production. One of Muyskens' students, Hide Shohara, made one of the earliest and clearest statements about "coarticulatory effects" in her 1932 dissertation titled *Genesis of Articulatory Movements of Speech (see also* Shohara, 1939). Two of Muyskens' other doctoral students, Harold Westlake and Martin Palmer, were major influences in examining and treating speech disorders of children with cerebral palsy. These individuals and their students strongly advocated a position that "speech was an overlaid function," a point to be discussed later in this chapter. The foundations for this point of view were in completed manuscript form by 1938, but publication was delayed until after World War II (Meader & Muyskens, 1950).

The arrival of Emil Froschels in this country in the mid-to-late 1930s also had great impact on this period's research and treatment of the dysarthrias, including adult dysarthrias. Froschels' view also was clearly neurobiologic, if you will, as evidenced in the English translation of his 1918 monograph *Childhood Language and Aphasia* (Rieber, 1980). Consider, as examples, the following chapter titles; "Reflections on the history of evolution of speech and the faults of an evolutionary approach," "The first stage of speech: Crying," "Babbling: The emergence of sensory components of the speech mechanism," and "The path from thinking to speaking."

The research of Raymond Stetson in this period also was a clear antecedent to present work on the motor control of speech and limb movements (Stetson, 1950). The work of Stetson and his colleagues, as well as Muyskens, formed the biologic bases for speech production in the literature for the first half of the 20th century.

1950–1970

The quantitative research in the years 1950-1970 emphasized differences between normal *group* performance and that of selected dysarthric subgroups. Examples included studies of parkinsonian dysarthria (c.f., Canter, 1963, 1965a, 1965b) and children with cerebral palsy (Hardy, 1964). For the most part, university coursework covered the dysarthrias in children (viz. cerebral palsy) and adults (as part of "Adult Neuropathologies of Speech and Language") in separate classes and many students may have missed the phylo-ontogenetic information of the former and the speech physiology data of the latter.

During this period, Eric Lenneberg (with *Biological Foundations of Language,* 1967) carried on the Muyskens tradition of accounting for evolutionary and biologic influences on the ontogeny of speech/language development and its disorders.

What seems clear to me from this short history is that the call for physiologic research of the dysarthrias near the end of this period (Darley, Aronson, & Brown, 1969a, 1969b; Hardy, 1966) was a logical extension of the preceding 50 years.

The 1970s

Research of dysarthria early in the 1970s was marked by physiologic studies of the "moment to moment" changes in muscle contractions and vocal tract movements (e.g., Kent, 1973; Logemann, Fisher, Boshes, & Blonsky, 1978; Netsell, 1971). Even these largely qualitative studies came rapidly to influence the clinical procedures of evaluation and treatment of individual dysarthric clients (e.g., Darley, Aronson, & Brown, 1975;

Netsell & Daniel, 1979; Rosenbek & LaPointe, 1978; Rubow, 1980). The establishment of an NIH Clinical Research Center at the University of Wisconsin in 1977 brought together an interdisciplinary team of basic and clinical scientists to study "neurogenic speech disorders." That work incorporates a combined systems analysis and a neurophysiologic approach to these problems and those studies are responsible, in large part, for the marked increase in our current understanding of the dysarthrias (e.g., Abbs, Hunker, & Barlow, 1983; Abbs & Kennedy, 1980; Barlow & Abbs, in press; Hunker & Abbs, this volume; Hunker, Abbs, & Barlow, 1982; Müller, Abbs, & Kennedy, 1981).

This physiologic research of the 1970s was almost entirely with adult dysarthrics and normal adult controls. Comparable studies of children with dysarthria are a clear research need, as will be elaborated below.

UNDERSTANDING THE DYSARTHRIAS

This section contains three major parts: understanding the (1) nervous system, (2) speech motor control, and (3) neuropathology. The intent is to show that this collective knowledge will enhance our understanding overall for individuals with dysarthria and optimal ways in which to treat their particular problems in gaining or regaining the ability to produce intelligible speech.

Understanding the Nervous System

Most clinical speech examinations represent a "time slice" view of the individual's speech patterns, with inferences to the underlying neuropathology. The review in this section emphasizes the continuously *evolving* nature of the nervous system, with special reference to the *distributed* and *interactive* neural mechanisms of speech and other behavior. Attention also is drawn to new data in neurotransmitter research and its relevance to understanding motor development in normal and disordered nervous systems.

Phylogeny. The study of phylogeny permits formulation of hypotheses based on the comparison of human evolution of brain/behavior characteristics with those of other animals. In comparing human and nonhuman primate vocalizations, it is assumed that there are neurobiologic and behavioral homologs, with the human advances representing a further differentiation and elaboration of the more primitive forms.

The current human nervous system has been depicted as a composite of reticular, limbic, and neocortical systems (MacLean, 1970; Moore, 1980; Mysak, 1976). The phylogenetically older parts (reticular and limbic) sufficed once to meet the survival needs of the organism, including communication, remaining with us to serve basic biologic responses (e.g., homeostasis, equilibrium, postural reactions, and feeding) and "affective/emotional" communications including crying, laughing, and facial expressions.

The neocortical system has evolved for expression of finer sensorimotor skills, including speech, music, and perhaps thought as well (Luria, 1981). The superior "analytic" skills (sensory, cognitive, and motor) of the human also are attributed to neocortical developments. The term "cortical" in "neocortical" can give the false impression that the "higher cortical functions" of man have their anatomic focus in the cerebral cortex. As described below, the neocortical system is distributed throughout the subcortical anatomy, including in the cerebellum. This helps explain why subcortical lesions in humans can have "analytic" as well as "affective/emotional" consequences for communication disorders (Brown, 1979; Kent, 1984).

In considering the human communication lessons to be learned from nonhuman primates, it's most advantageous when the latter have vocalizations in their repertoire that are "intentional" as well as "affective," where the former might be regarded as antecedents of human "analytic" speech. Even when this distinction is not clear as, for example in the squirrel monkey, the implications are provocative (c.f., Jurgens, 1979; Ploog, 1979, 1981). The squirrel monkey has a hierarchical organization of vocal control. At the top of this hierarchy is the cortex around the anterior cingulate cortex. This area seems to be responsible for the volitional initiation of phonation. The area's most important projections are those to the sensorimotor face cortex and to the periaqueductal region in the caudal midbrain. The face cortex, presumably responsible for the motor control of learned phonatory patterns, also projects to the periaqueduct, but has other pathways to brainstem nuclei. Motivational, or "innate," vocalizations survive lesions at higher centers and the cingulate region seems to exert only a facilitory or inhibitory influence on these calls. On the other hand, cingulate lesions disrupt the initiation of learned vocalization and face cortex lesions affect the motor coordination of these sound productions. These results point to separate pathways for the expression of innate and learned vocalizations and will be related inferentially to human vocalizations in the Understanding Neuropathology section below.

For a recent review of possible hemispheric differences in the organization of speech production see Kent (1984). MacNeilage (1983) is developing the hypothesis that the motor control for speech has evolved from the neural mechanisms used for bimanual coordination. The notion is that man first developed bimanual coordination by holding objects in the left hand and working on or manipulating them with the right hand. Rather than trying to control each hand separately from the contralateral hemisphere, MacNeilage further reasons that our ancestors developed control of bimanual coordination through one hemisphere, viz. the left. As a later development, we used many of these left brain neuronal connectivities (or similar homologs) for the motor control of speech.

Ontogeny. The ontogeny of human infant vocalization proceeds from the early innate expressions of need to those of "intended," learned vocalizations of *words* toward the end of their 1st year of life. The ontogeny of early word vocalizations is a subject of current research, as is the continuity/discontinuity issue of their origins in babbling and imitation (e.g., Bauer, Kent, & Murray, 1983; Oller, 1981). Neural maturation and vocal tract morphology undergo continuous changes through infancy and early childhood and parallel closely the motoric complexity of the developing vocalizations (Kent, 1981; Netsell, 1981). Neural maturation also progresses from brainstem to cortical regions in this period and, given the above discussion of phylogeny and separate pathways for innate and learned vocalizations, the natural history of speech motor development shows ontogeny to recapitulate phylogeny — at least in this regard.

The ontogeny of speech also qualifies speech production as a motor skill (Netsell, 1981; Wolff, 1979). It seems impossible, if not unnecessary, at this point to differentiate the development of speech motor skill from related skill development, viz. sensory, perceptual, and cognitive. If, as Luria (1981) contends, speech development in some way shapes cognitive development, then any distinction may be arbitrary. Regardless, delays in speech motor development may be more related to "learning disabilities" than has been apparent to date.

A tenet of ethology is that most behaviors have a "survival value," where the supporting anatomy and physiology have undergone and continue to undergo a continuous adaptation and further differentiation (Tinbergen, 1963). Vocalization, as a motor skill and expression of cognition/language, has evolved as a surival mechanism (communication), as a means of social interaction, and as a facilitator of thought. The vocalization reflects both the emotional and analytic state of the animal, where both speech and music contain this interaction in humans and express our most differentiated thoughts. Human "survival" and evolution obviously depend on the quality of these expressions.

The Role of Neurotransmitters. There have been several recent and major advances in understanding the contribution of neurotransmitters to mood, cognition, and activity (see reviews of Coyle, 1983; Johnston & Coyle, 1981).

Inter-neuronal communication is mediated to chemical neurotransmitters, which are released from the nerve terminal, diffuse across the synaptic cleft and interact with specific receptors on adjacent neurons. The development of the biochemical machinery for neurotransmission is closely linked to the functional maturation of the brain's neuronal circuitry. Components essential for neurotransmission (e.g., synthetic enzymes, endogenous neurotransmitters, re-uptake processes and receptors) serve as specific biochemical markers for neuronal systems. The appearance of and developmental increases in these markers during fetal and postnatal life occur with the cessation of neuronal replication and initiation of neuropil elaboration. Discrete groups of neurotransmitter-specific neurons develop according to different timetables, resulting in a shifting pattern of their relative influence in the maturing brain. (Johnston & Coyle, 1981, p.251)

Coyle (1983) emphasized four discrete neuronal groups, with differing loci in the nervous system, specific and often overlapping terminations, and different developmental courses. Also described are their differential effects on mood, cognition, and activity. Concerning the developmental course of these neurotransmitters, Coyle adds:

The noradrenergic pathways appear to be among the first to develop and their axons invade cerebral cortex during the very process of its formation. Thus, the noradrenergic input would appear to be an early and consistent source of innervation to the cerebral cortex and limbic systems. The serontonergic neurons develop somewhat later and appear to provide a more gradual developmental elaboration of their processes with the cortex and limbic system. The dopaminergic neurons exhibit a somewhat delayed innervation of the cortical limbic system and with the nigrostriatal dopaminergic projection appear to exhibit a gradual and progressive innervation over the first decade and one-half of postnatal life. Finally, the cholinergic projections to cerebral cortex develop in a delayed but rather abrupt fashion. This appears to occur during the first year of life in the human. (Coyle, 1983, p.2)

In general, the neurotransmitters provide a facilitative or suppressive effect on interneuronal communications, and these effects indirectly influence mood, cognition, and motor activity. With additional neurotransmitter research, we should better understand their influence on the development of speech motor control and its relationship to cognition as expressed through language. For example, Coyle (1983) mentioned that if autistic children do develop language, they do so around ages 4 to 5, a time when serotonin is known to sharply increase in the brain. Interestingly, this is a time when normal children rapidly increase the motoric complexity of their speech.

Further advances in understanding the developmental course and behavioral influences of each neurotransmitter should markedly influence our concepts of neuronal development and its contributions to emerging normal and pathologic behavior. Even the modest beginnings in this area have guided neurologists in pharmacologic treatments (see reviews in Ferrendelli, 1983; Rosenberg, 1983).

Understanding the Motor Control of Speech

Recent developments in our understanding of normal speech motor control have made an immediate impact on our ability to evaluate and treat the dysarthrias (e.g., see Abbs et al., 1983; Netsell, 1983; Rosenbek & LaPointe, 1978; Yorkston & Beukelman, 1981). As indicated previously, major advances have occurred in this area in the past decade (see review in Abbs & Cole, 1982). Earlier controversy regarding the (1) playing out of "overlearned" motor patterns versus (2) the use of peripheral afference to guide speech movements during their execution has resolved to some intermediate position.

Normal Adult Performance.

Spatial-Temporal Goals.—In attempting to generate the meaningful acoustics of speech, the speaker must bring the vocal tract to rather

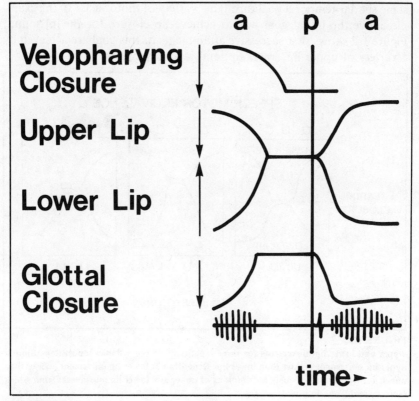

FIGURE 1-1

A schematic representation of the coordination of four structures in reaching a *spatial-temporal* goal. See text for discussion.

precise shapes at rather precise points in time. Figure 1-1 depicts one such *spatial-temporal goal* (Grillner, 1982; Lubker, 1982; Netsell, 1981). In producing the syllable [pɑ], a reasonably tight velopharyngeal closure must occur before lip release, and the glottis must be open before the lip release. This spatial-temporal precision occurs roughly in the time frame of 100 msec. Since the [p] production places no requirements on the tongue, this structure already is positioned (or is moving into position) for the [ɑ] sound. This is one example of movements "overlapping" one another, where one spatial-temporal goal is being achieved as another is being formed. This also is an example of the popular term "coarticulation." (See Hammarberg, 1982, for a thorough discussion of coarticulation.) Note also for the production of [ɑ] that the glottis must move rapidly from opening on the [p] to closing for the voicing of [ɑ].

Motor Equivalence.—Motor equivalence refers to the achievement of the same spatial-temporal goal through a variety of motor acts. In the example above,the initial goal was to achieve lip closure for the [p] sound. Figure 1-2 shows that successive attainments of this goal are achieved by a variety of upper lip, lower lip, and jaw movements.

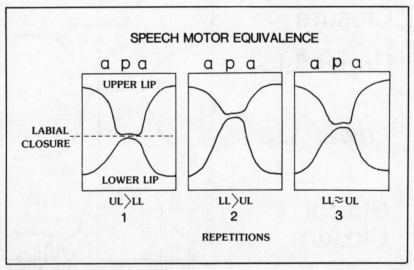

FIGURE 1-2
Upper and lower lip movements for three repetitions of the syllables [ɑpɑ]. Repetition 1: upper lip movement greater than lower lip. Repetition 2: lower lip movement greater than upper lip. Repetition 3: equal contributions of upper and lower lip movement (from Abbs, Gracco, and Cole, in press).

In achieving the vocal tract shape for [i], it appears necessary to reach only an "acoustically critical configuration" in the anterior oral cavity. Figure 1-3 compares the tongue shape for [i] where the jaw was free to move (solid lines) with its shape when the subject held a "bite-block" between the teeth, resulting in a fixed distance of 16 mm between the upper and lower incisors. With the bite-block in place, the tongue "automatically" reached the [i] goal, i.e., the speaker made these adjustments without any "conscious" effort to do so. Perkell and Nelson (1982) suggest that because most English vowels require quite distinct vocal tract shapes, that tongue positioning for repeated productions of the same vowel can vary by a few millimeters and still generate the requisite acoustics. Thus, whereas the bite-block studies reveal the precision of which we are capable, the precision used in "conversational speech" can be much less.

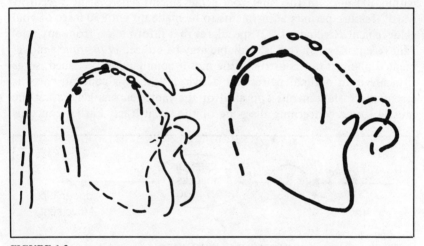

FIGURE 1-3
Mid-sagittal line drawings of the upper airway for [i] vowel productions. *Left side:* superimpositions of lip, tongue, pharynx, and jaw positions when the jaw was free to move (solid lines) and held in a fixed position (dashed lines). *Right side:* superimpositions of tongue shapes referenced to the jaw which show the extent of adjustment made with the tongue to achieve the tongue positions on the left.

Given these examples of "motor equivalence," it seems that the nervous system initially specifies the "goals" and leaves the details to be worked out — based, in part, on knowledge of the instantaneous state of the vocal tract. (See further discussion in Abbs & Kennedy, 1980.) How this might be accomplished is discussed in the next section.

Afferent Influences.—Consideration of "afferent influences" incorporates the concepts of "feedback" and "feedforward" (see Abbs & Cole, 1982; Evarts, 1982). These concepts are depicted in Figure 1-4. The *feedback* system is involved where information about the muscle action and movement is returned directly to the neural components regulating that action. *Feedforward* is used where information regarding the peripheral state is used to alter movements of other structures in order to achieve the particular spatial-temporal goal. In Figure 1-4, the "feedback" from the lower lip may be used in regulating its movement for the bilabial contact, while the same information is fed forward to be used in adjustments of the upper lip to effect the contact. Presumably, mechanisms such as these are operating in the trade-offs (motor equivalence) of the lips, as shown in Figure 1-3. Abbs and Cole (1982) hypothesize the "feedback" system to be useful in regulating movements within 100 msec of the final goal achievement; whereas the "feedforward" feature permits adjustments to be made up until 50 msec of goal achievement. Grillner (1982) speculates that information from any relevant receptor system that is available may be utilized *at the time* a movement is planned to "construct" the motor command to be issued, so as to achieve an optimal pattern of activity. With this concept, there is essentially instantaneous appraisal of the motoneurons generating the muscle forces concerning the state of the vocal tract. Earlier concerns

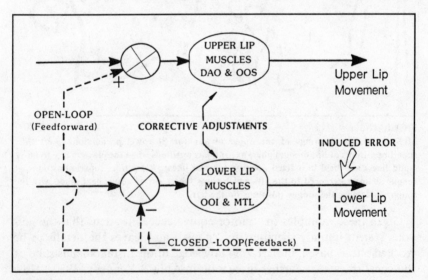

FIGURE 1-4
Schematic drawing to illustrate closed-loop (feedback) and open-loop (feedforward) mechanisms to the lips. See text for discussion (from Abbs and Gracco, in press).

that nervous system delays were too long for such fast modulations of motoneuron activity have been lessened by more recent theory and data (Abbs & Cole, 1982; Cole,1981).

Learning to talk. Little is known about the physiologic processes developed and used by normal children in learning the motor skills of speech. Knowledge of these processes is critical to understanding the dysarthrias of children (see reviews in Netsell, 1981, 1983).

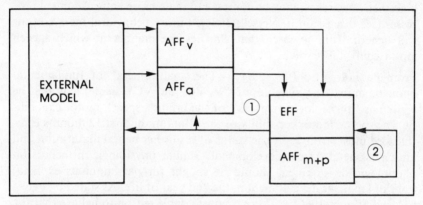

FIGURE 1-5
A block diagram of elements hypothesized to function in the acquisition of speech motor control. See text for discussion (from Netsell, 1981).

Afferent/Efferent Processes.—Figure 1-5 is a block diagram of afferent and efferent processes that have been hypothesized to operate as the infant/child is learning to talk. These ideas have been expressed elsewhere, including Hardy (1970), Meader and Muyskens (1950), Netsell (1981), and Rutherford (1967). It is hypothesized that the normal child learns to talk by listening, watching, and imitating an external model (e.g., a parent, caretaker, or other child). The model provides both auditory and visual afferent cues (AFF^a and AFF^v) which the child attempts to imitate with his or her own movements and vocalizations (shown as EFF, efferent). This EFF has two important consequences. First, it generates the auditory patterns that return to the ears of the model and child. The latter auditory feedback closes the important motor-auditory loop shown as (1) in Figure 1-5. Second, EFF creates feedback associated with the speech movements and postures (AFF^{m+p}) that the child pairs with his or her own auditory patterns. In essence, the child hears and "feels" his or her speech movements as they are being developed. This tight sensorimotor-auditory coupling presumably is the key to his refinement of the output (EFF) to approximate the external model. By this process, the child eventually develops internal representations in his nervous system of these sensorimotor actions.

It is not clear at this point that the child uses "conscious" control of speech movements in learning to talk. He or she may "unconsciously" develop control of speech movements in a manner similar to the way that adults "unconsciously" generate their speech movements. Intervention strategies that bring speech movement routines to a level of visual or kinesthetic awareness may be contrary to these more natural control processes (see discussion in Netsell, 1983). Future behavioral interventions will benefit from research that clarifies the manner in which speech motor control is learned.

From Phonology to Physiology.—The "naturalness" of fundamental phonetic units (e.g., syllables of CV, VC, and VCV shape) may best be viewed as "physiologic artifacts" of the infant's speech-motor capability. The speech motor capability of the infant in the first 12 months is influenced most strongly by the status of his or her neural maturation and musculoskeletal system development. Similar physiologic influences on phonologic development should be sought for parsimonious explanations of language development in the 2nd year of life. As stated by Peterson and Shoup (1966), "There is considerable reason to believe that the phonological aspects of speech are primarily organized in terms of the possibilities and constraints of the motor mechanism with which speech is produced." (p. 7)

Distributed systems and functions. Another important concept is that of *distributed* systems, especially in the neocortical system (see Mountcastle,

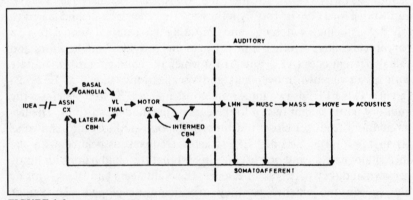

FIGURE 1-6
Diagrammatic representation of neural pathways, modules, and the musculoskeletal system hypothesized to be used in the motor control of speech. See text for discussion (from Netsell, 1982).

1978; & Figure 1-6). The concept here is that nuclei in different regions of the nervous sytem form interconnections to serve particular functions. Some functions share particular nuclei and pathways and not others. In addition, the "command neurons" for the different functions are located at different places in the nervous system. For example, breathing, sucking, chewing, and swallowing are thought to be driven by pacemaker neurons, or "pattern generators," located in the brainstem, whereas human speech motor control depends on more recently evolved neocortical structures.

UNDERSTANDING NEUROPATHOLOGY

In this section, an attempt is made to relate the previous discussions to neuropathology in the human nervous system, with particular reference to the neural mechanisms involved in the dysarthrias. Clearly, all that is written here is speculative, and as such, forms only the most rudimentary hypotheses for elaboration and experimental study.

Evolving and Interactive Systems

Reticular, limbic, and neocortical systems. Even though an earlier distinction was made between reticular, limbic, and neocortical systems, lesions often affect more than one. These systems are evolutionary in a phylogenetic and maturational sense; also, interactive and distributed throughout the nervous system in an anatomic and functional sense.

The reticular system, extending from lower to higher brainstem and including the basal nuclei, is both diffuse and specific in its organization and function. Lesions to respiratory centers, of course, are not compatible with life. Lesser lesions result in postural reactions (e.g., asymmetric tonic neck reflexes, righting reactions) that obligate the muscles and body parts to rather fixed postures and impair attempts at fine muscle contractions (Moore, 1980; Mysak, 1976, 1980). Patients with these problems reportedly gain relief from these symptoms through manipulations in the high cervical regions (c.f., Moore, 1980; Mysak, 1980). The reticular system also is believed to be "sensory oriented," in that multiple and specific sensory inputs collect there. One therapy rationale is aimed at differential stimulation of these sensory channels via peripheral nerves of differing diameter. (See discussion of M. Rood in Harris, 1969, 1971.)

Damage to the limbic system affects the individual's control of affect and the initiation of movement (see Brown, 1979; Kent, 1984). Uncontrolled bouts of crying or laughing often occur, as do vocalizations of a guttural or banal nature. What seems to be lacking is the engagement of the neocortical system for purposes of "ideational" speech. More severe involvement of limbic structures results in "akinetic mutism" (Brown,

1979; Kent, 1984). Recalling Ploog's work with squirrel monkeys discussed previously, lesions to the cingulate cortex left them unable to carry out "learned vocalizations," whereas their "affective" calls survived. Even neurologically normal speakers can have their speech nearly halted during moments of extreme anxiety. It is tempting to speculate that neurochemical thresholds in the limbic system can fluctuate, and, indeed are more "labile" in certain neuropathologies of the limbic system as well as during the more emotional movements of normal individuals.

The neocortical system, as the phylogenetically most advanced and maturationally last to develop, is believed responsible for all the human's most highly differentiated behaviors (including sensory, perceptual, motor, and cognitive). Cortical damage to the neocortical system (see Figure 1-6) can be massive outside of Broca's, Wernicke's, and the supplementary motor area — with intelligible speech preserved (Finger & Stein, 1982; Penfield & Roberts, 1959). Much smaller lesions at "summing points" for multiple inputs (e.g., Broca's area, motor sensory cortex, or cerebellum) can result in a dyspraxia or dysarthria. Brodal (1973), for example, believed his lesion was restricted to the right internal capsule and he reported problems with fine motor control of speech and writing that included errors of an apraxic nature, as well as dysarthria. This raises the issue as to whether or not apraxia of speech and dysarthria can appear separately when the neocortical system is damaged. Certainly, many apraxic speakers sound ataxic, and vice-versa. Considering also that apraxics have problems in constructing individual spatial-temporal goals (See Figure 1-1) as well as the serial ordering of those goals (See Fromm, 1981), the dyspraxic/dysarthric distinction becomes less clear in the neocortical system. The following discussion of evolving anterior and posterior systems may help to clarify some of the shared versus specialized systems for speech processes that, when impaired, yield symptoms we classify as dysarthric and dyspraxic, respectively.

Anterior versus posterior systems. Several authors, including Brown (1979), Mysak (1980), and Penfield and Roberts (1959), point to neuroanatomic and physiologic distinctions between an *anterior* and *posterior* system development that predominantly serve the production and perception components of speech, respectively. Brown reviews literature to support his view that anterior system damage results in several forms of expressive aphasia. He also points to the evolutionary and maturational progression of these systems through the reticular-to-limbic-to-neocortical developments, with the forms of speech/language disturbance falling on a continuum from "old brain" to "new brain." Brown (1979) also introduces the concept of an evolving "motor envelope."

The developing utterance issues out of a preliminary (limbic) cognition. Simultaneously, the action of the limbs proceeds outward towards objects in extrapersonal space. The diffuse, labile affect of the limbic level is derived into more differentiated partial expressions while consciousness of speech and action becomes increasingly more critical and acute.

From the point of view of the speech act, there is a progression from akinetic mutism, an inability to evoke or further realize the motor envelope of the speech act, through an attenuated form of transcortical motor aphasia, to agrammatism and finally Broca's aphasia proper. In this progression, the cognitive stage, as it is revealed in pathology, becomes increasingly more focused as it develops toward the final articulatory units.

The motor envelope contains the embryonic speech act together with its accompanying gestural and somatic motor elements. At this stage, the elements are only preconfigurative, bearing little resemblance to the performance (speech, gesture) to which they give rise.

At the point where the speech act differentiates out of this background organization, pathological disruption is characterized by a lack of spontaneous or conversational speech with good repetition. At times, naming and reading aloud are also spared. This constellation of findings has been termed *transcortical motor aphasia;* it is similar to the dynamic aphasia of Luria. In this syndrome, there is more than just a lack of spontaneous speech; nonspeech vocalizations and gestures are also reduced and there is often an inertia of behavior generally, which may suggest Parkinsonism. These "associated" symptoms all point to a common level or origin in the unfolding motor act; they are also a sign of its proximity to akinetic mutism.

This disorder reflects an involvement at the level of generation of an utterance, a speech act, without a disruption of the (potential) constituents of that act. This may concern the initiation of the utterance, its organization, and/or its differentiation from other motor elements at that level. Repetition aids in achieving this differentiation and in providing a configuration through which syntactic differentiation can occur. Naming is frequently preserved. The presence of an object may help to provide a structure through which this differentiation may occur. The presence of good naming in this disorder marks a transition to the next level, that of agrammatism, where there is also superior noun production.

The affective state of such patients is usually one of apathy or indifference. The apparent lack of emotional responsiveness is another feature indicating a link with cingulate gyrus disorders. However, the pathological anatomy is uncertain. At least it can be said that the preservation of repetition is not to be understood by the sparing of a repetition pathway; that is, it is not a transcortical defect (Brown, 1975). In many cases there is partial involvement of the left Broca area (Goldstein, 1915). I have described a case with subtotal destruction of Broca's area (Brown, 1975). On the other hand, the most frequent cause is probably occlusion of the anterior cerebral artery, which entails damage to the anterior cingulate gyrus, supplementary motor area and contiguous structures on the medial surface of the frontal lobe. Conceivably, the disorder may follow a left cingulate lesion as a partial form of the severe mutism with bilateral cingulate destruction. The association with supplementary motor area is now well-established. These contain limbic-derived neocortical zones. In any event, the correlation is either with limbic-transitional or *meso*cortex or with the next level in neocortical phylogenesis, generalized neocortex of the left frontal region.

As the speech act differentiates, the simpler and more global units of the utterance-to-be are the first to emerge. Along with the appearance of nouns and uninflected verbs, there is an unfolding into the forming utterance of the small grammatical or function words. The appearance of the functions is thus delayed to a level of individuation subsequent to that of holophrastic noun and verb production. Disorders at this stage are characterized by an incomplete differentiation of emerging syntactic units (agrammatism).

Conceivably, this disturbance can be conceptualized as an incomplete elaboration of a phrase structure type, with a premature appearance of representation at the noun and verb phrase level. If so, the nouns and verbs of agrammatic patients should not have precisely the same value as those same lexical units in normal speech. Certainly, agrammatics use nouns in a more diffuse, more propositional (holophrastic) way. Their difficulty in classifying nouns (Lhermitte et al., 1971) may reflect an attenuation of noun phrase differentiation. However, this is only a way of characterizing agrammatic language and may not reflect real psychological events. The preferential sparing of nouns and simple verbs in agrammatism may well have more to do with the initial use of these items as activity concepts, in relation to the cognitive mode of their acquisition. This is not to suggest that the agrammatic has a child's grammar; there is considerable evidence against this point of view. The evidence suggests, rather, that the young child's use of language in relation to activity may play a determining role in the psychological representation of these lexical items.(pp. 179-181)

This rather long excerpt from Brown (1979) reinforces a developing bias of this author that seems shared with Vygotsky, Luria, and the line of Russian thinking that apparently originated with Bereschew and Pavlov (see discussion in Meader & Muyskens, 1950, pp. 207-209). The thesis is that the ontogeny of the speech-motor act (i.e., the child's emerging expressions of thought through speech) is a prime determinant of cognitive development (including semantics and pragmatics), leaving "language," per se, with only the syntactic component, i.e., the agreed upon rules of order for the emergence and differentiation of thought (also see Robinson, 1975). Surely the details of Brown's predictions will be revised as the appropriate clinical and neurobiologic data become available. Nonetheless, Brown's concept of the evolving "motor envelope" represents to me a beginning set of biologic-behavioral hypotheses about these processes — with a clear pointer to phylo-ontogenetic determinants of speech and thought as well as the neurosymptomatology that will appear according to the age of the patient and the locus of the lesion. Brown's additional points are that the lesion usually must be bilateral to be of clinical significance and that subcortical lesions are more devastating than cortical lesions.

Distributed Functions and Restricted Lesions

The studies of Darley et al. (1969a; 1969b) provided a springboard for physiology studies in the 1970s. Five perceptually distinct forms of dysarthria were identified, and hypotheses were formed regarding their pathologic neuroanatomy and neurophysiology. Netsell (1982) reviewed the physiology studies of the 1970s concerning flaccid, ataxic, and parkinsonian dysarthria. In this section, particular emphasis is given to the effects of lesions at various levels of the brainstem on speech function. These lesions and associated speech disturbances give further clues about the organization of speech neural mechanisms and point to the need for refinement as well as elaboration of current classifications of the dysarthrias.

For this discussion, the brainstem is defined as the medulla oblongata, pons, and midbrain (Warwick & Williams, 1973). In general, lesions restricted to the cranial nerves and cell bodies yield the classic signs of "flaccid dysarthria" (Darley et al., 1969a, 1969b), but even this "neurologic truism" may have exceptions. Bratzlavsky and vander Eecken (1977) believed their seven patients had undergone altered synaptic organization of the facial nucleus following facial nerve regeneration during recovery from Bell's palsy. The earlier flaccid signs were replaced by a "hemifacial hypertonia." So-called "irritative" brainstem lesions that act on the inputs of the cranial nerve nuclei also can yield symptoms of hypertonicity (Jankovic & Patel, 1983).

Congenital or acquired lesions in the lower brainstem (medulla and pons) that involve the reticular core result in hypertonic postures and reactions in the head, neck, torso, and limbs (Mysak, 1976; 1980). Netsell and Daniel (1979) speculated that their client showed "flaccid" signs in the orofacial system and "spastic" limbs as trauma residuals affecting the lower and upper motoneurons of the lower brainstem for the cranial and spinal motor systems, respectively.

Studies of the "locked in syndrome" (LiS) point to other restricted motor pathways of the rostral brainstem, viz. the rostral pons and cerebral peduncles at the lower midbrain (see reviews in Bauer, Gerstenbrand, & Rumpl, 1979; Bauer, Gerstenbrand, & Hengl, 1980). In its pure form, LiS permits no movement other than vertical deflections of the eyes. LiS patients signal with their eyes that they have sensory as well as considerable cognitive function, including one case where the above-average cognition has been preserved for 12 years (Cappa & Vignolo, 1982). More typically, the LiS is incomplete and the patients vocalize to emotional stimuli and show limited movements of the limbs (Bauer et al., 1979; Bauer et al., 1980).

These varieties of LiS suggest that limbic and perhaps reticular pathways also are involved. Although rare, recovery from LiS does occur (McCusker, Rudick, Honch, & Griggs, 1982). McCusker et al. documented four such cases and the early return of function did not predict a better overall recovery. All four patients were believed to have ventral pontine infarcts. Two of these cases demonstrated trismus (tonic spasms of the jaw muscles). If the other two cases had "subclinical" trismus, it could be hypothesized that trismus resulted from upper motoneuron lesions of the trigeminal system as well as cranial nuclei below the pons. This could account for flaccid facial muscles and hypertonic, or "spastic" muscles whose cranial nuclei were inferior to the lesion. Alternatively, only muscles with spindles might show "spasticity" (see discussion in Barlow & Abbs, in press).

Bauer, Prugger, and Rumpl (1982) report three cases of LiS demonstrating stimulus-evoked "oral automatisms." Although sucking and chewing movements never occurred spontaneously, these could be evoked with oral or perioral stimulation. The authors speculate that complete systems for sucking and chewing exist in the brainstem that can be evoked in the absence of cortical input.

Bilateral lesions involving corticobulbar and corticospinal pathways in the midbrain may yield the purer forms of "pseudobulbar palsy." Lesions at this level may produce "weakness" and "spasticity" due to the "direct" and "indirect" cortical projections, respectively (Darley et al., 1975), and the pathologic crying and laughter due to limbic system damage. Higher lesions involving thalamus and cortex are complicated by aphasia, apraxia, or both (Brown, 1979). Indeed, as suggested by Brodal (1973), unilateral involvement at the internal capsule may yield not only a dysarthria, but a dyspraxia as well. More discussion of Brodal's case is found later in Treating the Dysarthrias.

The natural course of recovery following traumatic midbrain lesions offers further clues regarding the motor organization of speech. Vogel and von Camon (1982) described voice recovery in eight patients with severe head trauma and sequelae that were hypothesized to result from compression of midbrain structures caused by cerebral swelling. An initial stage of mutism was accompanied by "affective" vocalizations (groaning, sighing, laughing, and crying) and involuntary coughs. The patients could produce no vocalization or other movement at will.

Of the six patients who were tested with the short form of the Token Test, "an aphasic disorder could be excluded." The mutism was followed by a "whispery stage," lasting 1 to 3 weeks, in which "phonologically relevant movements appeared that were impaired in the majority of patients" (p. 153). In some patients, expiratory, and inspiratory breathing patterns alternated from one syllable to the next, and "coughing, throat clearing, etc. could not be produced at will during this stage" (p. 153). There was a 2 to 3 week transition stage from whispered to "constant voiced production," where voice production was variable, breathy, and reduced in loudness. Once a constant voice was achieved, all types of vocalization could be produced at will. "An appropriate loudness level during conversational speech was the first vocal parameter to reach normal limits" (p. 154). The remaining voice problems included a "limited ability to regulate pitch and the reduced pitch range," and, the development of a "tense voice." The latter resembled "spastic dysphonia" and was believed to reflect a compensatory, overcontraction of laryngeal adductor muscles. Commenting on some of the same patients, von Cramon (1981) noted:

> During the transition between mutistic stage and the reappearance of verbal utterances patients produced central vowels and slides only, the first being "ja" (yes). Opening but also rounding and spreading of the lips were markedly restricted. As soon as consonants could be differentiated, patients showed a tendency to shift places of articulation posteriorly. An analysis of the manner of articulation revealed that the patients were not able to produce, and later to maintain, occlusions or stable constrictions...The most salient feature, however, was the impaired motor control of the tongue tip...The motor disturbance of the front part of the tongue persisted as long as the patients were observed. (p. 803)

Considering our earlier discussion of the lesion studies of the squirrel monkeys, the vocalization recovery of these midbrain patients shows several parallels. As emotional vocalizations were possible in the mutistic stage, von Cramon (1981) assumed the periaqueductal grey had been spared. The general course of voice and speech recovery also recapitulated the normal acquisition of speech motor skill in normal infants and children, giving some credence to von Cramon's hypothesis that "the most likely explanation is that traumatic mutism is caused by a temporal inhibition of neural activity within the brainstem vocalization system."

Shared vs. Specialized Neuronal Mechanisms

Meader and Muyskens (1959) believed that speech motor functions were phylo- and ontogenetic differentiations of the more primitive functions of sucking, chewing, and swallowing. "Thus, we see that specific vegetative structures and functions arose through a process of fragmentation of the simpler peristaltic structures and functions. These newer functions formed the matrix from which the speech movements emerged" (p. 243).

Vocal tract movements for vowel and consonants were said to have emerged from fragmentation of the peristaltic wave (Meader & Muyskens, 1950; Shohara, 1932). The supporting data were drawn from X-ray similarities of tongue shapes during vowel productions and segments of the swallowing act (Shohara, 1932). Speech was said to be an "overlaid function" on these vegetative functions. Treatments evolved from this view, including a hierarchical scheme that sucking, swallowing, and chewing, were determinants of and prerequisites for speech (e.g., see Crickmay, 1977; Fawcus, 1969). Among the clinical observations that reinforce the "overlaid" hypothesis are (1) speech is almost always severely involved when swallowing is a problem; (2) speech improves with improvement in swallowing; (3) chewing and swallowing can be normal and speech severely dysarthric; and (4) the act of simultaneous chewing and speaking is reported to improve speech when attempts to speak without chewing are unsuccessful.

All the necessary neuronal machinery for these vegetative acts is located within the brainstem. Cortical motoneurons may participate in certain aspects of chewing, but they are not necessary. The hypothesis is that sucking and swallowing are phylogenetically older and controlled by reticulo-limbic structures of the brainstem. Chewing has evolved more recently and, with the appearance of teeth, may require sensorimotor interactions of the tongue and jaw that are antecedents to tongue-jaw neuronal mechanisms used in speaking. Our ancestors undoubtedly vocalized while chewing and heard more differentiated sound patterns from the tongue movements. These "new sounds" may have become a way to signal more discrete units of "meaning" in their communication and may have been the origins of tongue movements for speech. Studies of tooth eruption and the differentiation of tongue movements for speech in individual infants may show a similar progression.

The point of the foregoing is to suggest that the neuronal mechanisms for speech are not simply "overlaid" on those of vegetation any more than the neocortical system is "overlaid" on the limbic or reticular systems. All oromotor functions are impaired when shared or adjacent neuronal structures are damaged (e.g., cranial nerves or cranial nuclei). Damage to brainstem pathways can interrupt fibers of all afferent-efferent systems. The alternative to the "overlaid" hypothesis is, that with the emergence of the neocortical system, the human sends unique commands to the lower motoneurons for speech and other fine motor skills. These may or may not be the same cell bodies and axons activated during vegetative acts. Regardless, both the patterns of activation and loci of the "command neurons" are specialized and differential for the motor acts of speech versus sucking, chewing, and swallowing.

Recovery from Brain Injury

Recent reviews reveal that many brain injured patients can show remarkable improvements beyond the usual 2 years, and various forms of treatment (including behavioral therapies) can facilitate the natural recovery processes (Bach-y-Rita, 1980; Finger & Stein, 1982). Wall's summary (1980) draws attention to the many factors involved in recovery and suggests factors that can and cannot be assumed to be of influence.

We can begin with the fact that those who survive brain damage show a surprising degree of recovery. No doubt some of this recovery is to be attributed to readjustments of the blood vessels and other factors on which the brain depends. However, some degree of recovery is seen even when there is known permanent destruction of parts of the nervous system. Certain mechanisms cannot be proposed to explain the recovery. Brain cells in the adult do not divide to reproduce new cells. Nerve fibers cut across in the central nervous system do not regenerate as they do in the periphery. Certain suggestions to explain recovery are rejected as being unhelpful and mystical since they do not specify what it is that has changed during recovery. Words such as shock, diaschisis and redundancy are not useful. There is no doubt that the patient learns to substitute alternative mechanisms for those he has lost just as a blind man develops his skills of hearing and feeling and just as an amputee extends the repertoire of his remaining limbs. Beyond this crucial learning there are signs of unlearned readjustments within the brain. Nerve cells show a type of homeostasis so that if they lose part of their input, they adjust their excitability to capture fully the excitatory effects of their remaining input. Where nerve fibers degenerate, the nearby intact fibers have an ability to sprout and occupy the site left vacant by the degenerated fibers. Beyond this sprouting mechanism there are large numbers of normally ineffective nerve connections which may become active if the dominant inputs are out of action. It is proposed that the connections laid down in the embryo are more diffuse than those actually used in the adult brain. The stage of maturation involves partly destruction of the "incorrect" connections and partly their suppression. If some nervous connections are destroyed in the adult, suppressed connections may become depressed. This is not necessarily a good thing: the substituted connections may bring in nonsense information which the recovering nervous system cannot handle. Sprouting and the unmasking of ineffective connections offers the possibility of new connections after brain damage, but we need to know much more about these processes so that we can guide them to useful ends rather than towards further disorganization (pp. 103–104).

TREATING THE DYSARTHRIAS

Incorporating much of the above discussion, suggestions and hypotheses are offered for consideration in treating the individual with dysarthria. It will be obvious that these are matters for research, rather than data-based clinical procedures or recommendations.

Factors Influencing Treatment Outcome

In considering treatment for the individual with dysarthria, several factors influence the eventual level of speech production skill that can be expected. These factors include the (1) neurologic status and history, (2) age, (3) "automatic" adjustments, (4) treatment effects, (5) personality and intelligence, and (6) support systems.

Neurologic status and history. The overriding factor influencing motor performance, in general, and speech production, in particular, would seem to be the location, extent, and underlying neuropathology of the lesion or lesions. As reviewed above, bilateral subcortical or brainstem lesions seem most devastating and least reversible. Less massive lesions to cortical aspects of the neocortical system offer a better prognosis, and even unilateral left brain lesions sparing subcortical structures have optimistic outcomes. The issue of neuropathology is most critical in cases of degenerative disease, e.g., amyotrophic lateral sclerosis, or dystonia musculorum deforms. Even in these cases, however, the deterioration can be gradual over a number of years and both biomedical and behavioral treatments can help in maintaining communication skills. The human nervous system has remarkable capabilities to work around or through lesions. Even though lesions place certain limits on performance, only the most severe (viz. those causing an unremitting mutism) would appear to be unresponsive to therapeutic intervention.

The individual's neurologic history also is an obvious consideration. The adult with a developmental dysarthria (e.g., cerebral palsy) has different needs in terms of speech motor learning than one who was neurologically normal before insult. A young school-aged child with head injury who was progressing normally would seem to need a different treatment program from a youngster with a history of developmental disability. Even though knowledge of the premorbid history is critical, it often is overlooked or unavailable.

Age. Given the course of neural maturation just outlined, persons experiencing neurologic insults following early but incomplete development of the neocortical system (say, perhaps after age 2 or 3) might be expected to have, or to develop, better speech motor skills than those lesioned earlier. Lenneberg (1968) reports that many infants with cortical and lesser subcortical lesions appear symptom-free until the 1st or 2nd year when they "grow into" the lesion. The implication is that intact reticulo-limbic systems can support the more innate early motor skills. Problems with learned motor skills become evident as the neocortical system fails to develop. Younger children have a better chance to "grow out of" or "around" their lesions than adults, presumably because the children's developing neuronal connectivities are more "plastic." Elderly patients, on the other hand, would seem most negatively affected by the age variable since their nervous systems are deteriorating as a natural process. However, a recent case study of an 83-year-old who used EMG feedback to relieve chronic facial spasm illustrates that even the severely involved, geriatric patient can benefit from carefully planned treatment (Rubow, Rosenbek, Collins, & Celesia, in press).

"Automatic" adjustments. In response to a lesion, the individual makes a variety of "automatic" adjustments; some are adaptive and others are maladaptive. Some are intended and others are unintended, reactive, or "obligatory" as a consequence of the neuropathology. A major task for the clinician is to identify these "automatic" adjustments during the evaluation period; incorporating those that are useful in developing or restoring speech and removing or minimizing those that are not.

Treatment effects. Obviously the selection of treatments (whether medical, physical, behavioral, or some combination) can affect speech production. Unfortunately, the selection of treatments usually reflects the educational and experience biases of the clinician as opposed to the most efficacious treatment. Fortunately, the adaptive and robust nature of the nervous system allows most clients to improve their speech, regardless of clinician bias. In the absence of data on comparative treatments, it is this writer's opinion that almost any speech therapy for a dysarthric client is helpful; few *speech* therapies are directly harmful; and the "whatever works" approach will continue to dominate most therapies until we learn more about the physiology and neuropathophysiology of speech. Basic and clinical researchers must join in these studies of the speech mechanism and the differential response of the dysarthric client to various treatments.

A related problem is that often the combined efforts of the physician, speech clinician, and occupational and physical therapists are not optimally coordinated. Even when speech appears not to be a primary concern, the speech clinician must know the helpful or deleterious effects on speech of the treatments provided by the other disciplines. For example, bilateral ventrolateral thalamic surgery can relieve tremor, rigidity, or dystonia in the limbs and leave the patient with a persistent, often severe, dysarthria (Cooper, 1969).

Personality and intelligence. A major influence on the eventual intelligibility of speech for the dysarthric client is his or her premorbid personality and intelligence. In my experience, the more dominant factor is personality and those who were optimistic and purposeful before injury have a clear advantage over those who were not. Establishing the premorbid intelligence is important in considering treatment objectives and outcomes when there is cause to suspect subnormal levels prior to injury.

Support systems. The ongoing treatment and carry-over of skills is enhanced for the brain-injured patient when there are "significant others" in his or her life and the prospects for making contributions to society, however modest, are realistic. Again, in my experience, these individuals have a much better prognosis for maintaining intelligible speech or optimizing use of augmentative communication aids. For a review of augmentative communication systems, see Linebaugh, Baird, Baird, and Armour (1983).

The Effects of Treatment for the Dysarthrias

Earlier beliefs that most unintelligible dysarthrics were restricted to this condition for life have been dispelled for the most part by a number of case studies. Whereas recent advances in neurochemical treatments are more obvious (e.g., see Coyle, 1983), those in clinical speech treatments seem less well recognized by other disciplines. Most new colleagues I meet in medicine (viz. neurology, pediatrics, rehabilitation medicine, and otolaryngology) or neuroscience are unaware that even severely impaired dysarthrics can respond to behavioral interventions. Even many speech clinicians are unaware of behavioral interventions or are unprepared to be helpful with severe cases.

A neurophysiologic emphasis. Even though the obvious goal is to improve speech intelligibility, acceptability, or both, the most efficacious demonstrations of change are accompanied by physiologic or neurophysiologic recordings. These recordings are imperative in attempting to normalize a subsystem (e.g., respiratory) when no immediate increase in intelligibility is to be expected (e.g., see Abbs, Hunker, & Barlow, 1983; Netsell & Daniel, 1979; Rosenbek & LaPointe, 1978). Perhaps the most powerful paradigm for the immediate future will be case studies that incorporate clinical (neurologic and speech), neurochemical, and physiologic or neurophysiologic data. For an example of this in the neurology literature, see Chadwick, Hallett, and Harris, (1977). Concerning the clinical speech data, it is imperative to document changes in speech intelligibility or acceptability.

Perceptual and acoustic documentation of speech changes. Perceptual ratings of speech intelligibility are most valid when evaluated by listeners unfamiliar with the speaker or the subject matter (context) of the spoken material. This is easily achieved by having uninvolved staff members rate edited samples of the client's conversation. Documenting the contributing changes in articulation skill, speaking rate, and so on, can be done by the speech specialists (e.g., using the rating scales of Darley et al., 1975) and/or measurements of speech acoustics (e.g., see Weismer, this volume; Weismer & Cariski, in press).

Choice of treatments.   The treatments that have persisted over the years have been based upon particular neurophysiologic hypotheses (e.g., neuro-developmental treatment, neuromuscular facilitation, the motokinesthetic method). Treatment procedures and their sequencing are developed from these hypotheses, but very little (if any) behavioral or physiologic data are available to demonstrate the effectiveness of a given procedure, or its advantage over an alternative procedure. In the absence of these data, it is difficult to recommend a given treatment at the expense of another. Many clinicians are forced to develop an eclectic approach that incorporates features of different theories or methods. Recent advances in physiologic recordings during speech should be helpful in remedying this situation.

Lessons from Brodal.   Brodal's (1973) reflections on his recovery following a stroke suggest that almost all the treatments offered him were of some value. He also was impressed that a right hemisphere lesion had disturbing effects on motor control of same (ipsilateral) body side. No clinical evidence of aphasia was found, but he described problems with "short term memory" and apraxic-like errors in writing and speaking. During speech, "sometimes a word was skipped or a syllable, especially at the end of a sentence, or two small words were incorrectly fused" (p. 686). He hypothesized that the dysarthria, which persisted for at least 10 months, resulted from the asymmetry of bilateral innervation, and destruction of ipsilateral corticofugal fibers, including corticopontine fibers which he estimated to outnumber pyramidal fibers by approximately 19 to 1. Brodal also speculated the dysarthria was related to a disturbance of cerebellar influence, via ponto-cerebello-thalamic connections. As Brodal points out, only autopsy will verify that no left hemisphere lesion existed and that his lesion was restricted to the right internal capsule. Regardless, his thoughts about lost and recovered functions following stroke are among the most informative ever written. Even though the paragraphs below relate to his problems in regaining use of the extremities, the parallels in restoring the motor control for speech appear to be strong.

The Value of Passive Movements.—In addition to helping maintain a full range of motion in the joints, Brodal felt the passive movements of the physical therapist helped him initiate and direct the desired movement.

> Subjectively, it was clearly felt as if the sensory information produced by the passive movement helped the patient to "direct" the "force of innervation" through the proper channels...It may well be that there are subtle neurophysiological mechanisms involved in this "facilitation" of movements. From introspection it appears, however, that the subjective information about the movement to be executed, its range and goal, is an essential factor. The phenomenon is probably parallel to the learning of all motor skills. Among an original multitude of more or less haphazard movements, the correct ones are recognized as such by means of the sensory information they feed back to the central nervous system, and this information is later used in selecting the correct movements in the further training. (p. 678)

Skilled Movements.—Brodal illustrated his loss of skilled movement by describing problems in tying his bow tie, a skill he had used daily for some 40 years.

> The appropriate finger movements were difficult to perform with sufficient strength, speed and coordination, but it was quite obvious to the patient that the main reason for failure was something else.
>
> Under normal conditions the necessary numerous small delicate movements had followed each other in the proper sequence almost automatically, and the act of tying when first started had proceeded without much conscious attention. Subjectively the patient felt as if he had to stop because "his fingers did not know the next move." He had the same feeling as when one recites a poem or sings a song and gets lost. The only way is to start from the beginning. It was felt as if the delay in the succession of movements (due to paresis and spasticity) interrupted a chain of more or less automatic movements. Consciously directing attention to the finger movements did not improve the performance; on the contrary it made it quite impossible. (p. 679)

Force of Innervation.—A final problem of Brodal's that may relate to speech rehabilitation was with what he termed the "force of innervation."

> It was a striking and repeatedly made observation that the force needed to make a severely paretic muscle contract is considerable. The expression of this force in this connection refers to what one, for the lack of a better expression, might call force of innervation. Subjectively, this is experienced as a kind of mental force, a power of will. In the case of a muscle just capable of being actively moved, the mental effort needed was very great. The greater the degree of paresis of such a muscle, the greater was the mental effort needed to make it contract and to oppose voluntarily even a very weak counter-force. On the other hand, only a slight mental effort was needed to bring about a fairly good contraction of a muscle able to work with about half or a little less of its full force. (p. 677)

Speech Therapy.—Brodal did not mention receiving any formal speech therapy. It may be that his speech recovery, which took at least 10 months, was essentially due to natural recovery. It may be that his recovery would have been accelerated by certain behavioral procedures. For example, the use of lip force or EMG feedback might have been helpful in the early stages of weakness, where movement could not be "willed." This might have allowed him to re-establish afferent-to-efferent relationships earlier, as well as initiate muscle contractions more rapidly. Brodal felt the loss of sequencing skilled movements was not due simply to problems with strength, speed, and coordination; rather he pointed to the loss of "automaticity" in sequencing. Given earlier discussion in this chapter about the importance of instantaneous afference in the regulation, if not construction, of individual spatial-temporal goals, it is hypothesized that the "getting lost" in a sequence is caused by a reduction in speed of movement associated with individual goal achievement. That is, the quantity and quality of afference generated during the slow movements may be "confusing" or insufficient for achievement of the intended goal and the speaker does not move on "automatically" to the next goal.

In other cases of severe dysarthria, the force or EMG feedback work could be tried (1) when no speech was possible, (2) as an adjunct to speech initiation, or (3) when attempting movements for individual spatial-temporal goals.

Shared and specialized mechanisms. The extent to which the neural mechanisms of speech share the phylo- or ontogenetic mechanisms used for sucking, chewing, or swallowing is a matter for further research. Feeding therapy undoubtedly helps some children to feed better, and may even facilitate vocalization development (Morris, 1980). The "inhibition" of detrimental postural reactions, careful presentation of graded orofacial stimuli, and other means to counteract "primitive behavior" may all facilitate speech development. But, it does not necessarily follow that these are antecedents to, or prerequisites for, the neural connectivities developed for or used in speaking. In the absence of data, perhaps a conservative blend of theory and practice is most appropriate in the clinic. For example, consider treating a presumed antecedent behavior when the more recently evolved or acquired behavior is not present. When the antecedents are believed to be necessary prerequisites, consider treating the highest level available of the desired skill (speech) simultaneous with the available level of the antecedent behavior. For example, "chewing therapy" may facilitate speech not because it's a phylo- or ontogenetic determinant, but because (1) it generates afferent consequences of oromotor movements (when speech cannot), (2) it forces speech motor equivalence during the chewing act, and/or because (3) the afference generated during chewing engages neuronal connections that are common to both chewing and speech.

Consider the thesis that speech and other fine motor skills are a "quantum leap" beyond earlier structure and function. This "quantum leap" is not a discontinuity in evolution, but an acceleration that yields clear advantages in adapting to the present environment and shaping its future. Clinically, this line of thinking might translate to the following question: Would you ask Philippe Entremont (classical painist), in attempting to regain the motor skill of piano playing, to begin at any skill level *below* the most advanced that he could demonstrate during testing?

Carryover from Clinic to the Outside

The transfer of the speaking skills obtained in the clinic to "real world" situations is a much needed area of research. The incorporation of "real world" speaking skills, situations, and strategies for maintaining them need to be introduced in clinic work at the earliest appropriate time.

EPILOGUE

In many (if not most) respects, Luria encompassed 25 years ago the ideas presented in this neurobiologic view of the dysarthrias. It is of interest that toward the end of his life he was planning to study the subcortical influences of speech, language, and thought, with special emphasis on neurochemical mechanisms.

The basic theme of this chapter has been that nothing is *static* — not the organism, its behavior, or its response to lesion or treatment. A neurobiologic view is at once converging and diverging. The *convergence* is seen in the neurologic reductionism to understand the organism's behavior in terms of its present (and past) structure and function. The *divergence* is in the brain and behavior of the organism, where continued differentiation of thought and elaboration of the nervous system remind us of our potential for growth. Little has been said of so-called "psychological functions" because they are believed to be biologic ones not yet understood.

NOTE

---

[1]These three areas represent the basic tenets of ethology, a discipline that Tinbergen (1963) stated was basically the study of the biology of behavior.

REFERENCES

Abbs, J., & Cole, K. Consideration of bulbar and suprabulbar afferent influences upon speech motor coordination and programming. In S. Grillner, B. Lindblom, J. Lubker, & A. Persson (Eds.), *Speech motor control.* New York: Pergamon, 1982.

Abbs, J.H., & Gracco, V.L. Sensorimotor actions in the control of multimovement speech gestures. *Trends in neuroscience,* in press.

Abbs, J.H., Gracco, V.L., & Cole, K.J. Control of multimovement coordination: sensorimotor mechanisms in speech motor programming. *Journal of Motor Behavior,* in press.

Abbs, J.H., & Kennedy, J. Neurophysiological processes of speech movement control. In N. Lass, J. Northern, D. Yoder, & L. McReynolds (Eds.), *Speech, language, and hearing.* Philadelphia: W.B. Saunders, 1980.

Abbs, J., Hunker, C.J., & Barlow, S.M. Differential speech motor subsystem impairments with suprabulbar lesions: Neurophysiological framework and supporting data. In W. Berry, (Ed.), *Clinical dysarthria.* San Diego: College-Hill Press, 1983.

Bach-y-Rita. *Recovery of function: Theoretical considerations for brain injury rehabilitation.* Baltimore: University Park Press, 1980.

Barlow, S.M., & Abbs, J.H. Orofacial fine motor control impairments in congenital spasticity: Evidence against hypertonus related performance deficits. *Journal of Neurology,* in press.

Bauer, G., Gerstenbrand, F., & Rumpl, E. Varieties of the locked-in syndrome. *Journal of Neurology,* 1979, *221,* 77-91.

Bauer, G., Gerstenbrand, F., & Hengl, W. Involuntary motor phenomena in the locked-in syndrome. *Journal of Neurology,* 1980, *223,* 191-198.

Bauer, H., Kent, R., & Murray, A. *Ethologic perspectives on first word development.* Paper presented to the Midwest Regional Animal Behavior Meeting, St. Louis, 1983.

Bauer, G., Prugger, M., & Rumpl, E. Stimulus evoked oral automatisms in the locked-in syndrome. *Archives of Neurology,* 1982, *39,* 435-436.

Bratzlavsky, M., & vander Eecken, H. Altered synaptic organization in facial nucleus following facial nerve regeneration: An electrophysiological study in man. *Annals of Neurology,* 1977, 2, 71-73.

Brodal, A. Self-observations and neuro-anatomical considerations after a stroke. *Brain* 1973, *96,* 675-694.

Brown, J. Language representation in the brain. In H. Steklis & M. Raleigh, (Eds.), *Neurobiology of social communication in primates: An evolutionary perspective.* New York: Academic Press, 1979.

Brown, J. On the neural organization of language: Thalamic and cortical relationships. *Brain and Language,* 1975, *2,* 18-30.

Canter, G. J. Speech characteristics of patients with Parkinson's disease: I. Intensity, pitch, and duration. *Journal of Speech and Hearing Disorders,* 1963, *28,* 221-229.

Canter, G. J. Speech characteristics of patients with Parkinson's disease: II. physiological support for speech. *Journal of Speech and Hearing Disorders,* 1965, *30,* 44-49.

Canter, G. J. Speech characteristics of patients with Parkinson's disease: III. Articulation, diadochokinesis, and overall speech adequacy. *Journal of Speech and Hearing Disorders,* 1965, *30,* 217-224.

Cappa, S., & Vignolo, L. Locked-in syndrome for 12 years with preserved intelligence. *Annals of Neurology,* 1982, *11,* 545.

Chadwick, D., Hallett, M., & Harris, R. Clinical, biochemical and physiological factors distinguishing myoclonus responsive to 5-hydroxytryptophan, tryptophan plus a monoamine oxidase inhibitor and clonazepam. *Brain,* 1977, *100,* 455-487.

Cole, K. *An empirical re-evaluation of minimum voluntary afferent-to-efferent pathway latencies in the orofacial system.* Unpublished master's thesis, University of Wisconsin, Madison, 1981.

Cooper, I. *Involuntary movement disorders.* New York: Harper & Row, 1969.

Coyle, J. *Neurotransmitter systems in psychotic and cognitive behavior.* Paper presented to the Symposium on Developmental Disabilities V: Autism and Related Disorders of Communication. Johns Hopkins Medical Center, Baltimore, 1983.

Cramon, von D. Traumatic mutism and the subsequent reorganization of speech functions. *Neuropsychologia,* 1981, *19,* 801-805.

Crickmay, M. *Speech therapy and the bobath approach to cerebral palsy.* Springfield, IL: C.C. Thomas, 1977.

Darley, F., Aronson, A., & Brown, J. Differential diagnostic patterns of dysarthria. *Journal of Speech and Hearing Research,* 1969, *12,* 246-269.

Darley, F. L., Aronson, A. E. & Brown, J. R. Clusters of deviant speech dimensions in the dysarthrias. *Journal of Speech and Hearing Research,* 1969, *12,* 462-496.

Darley, F., Aronson, A., & Brown, J. *Motor speech disorders.* Philadelphia: Saunders, 1975.

Evarts, E. Analogies between central motor programs for speech and for limb movements. In S. Grillner, B. Lindblom, J. Lubker, & A Persson (Eds.), *Speech motor control,* New York: Pergamon Press, 1982.

Fawcus, B. Oropharyngeal function in relation to speech. *Developmental Medicine and Child Neurology,* 1969, *11,* 556-560.

Ferrendelli, J. Neuropharmacology. Shortcourse presented to the 35th meeting of the American Academy of Neurology, San Diego, 1983.

Finger, S, & Stein, D. *Brain damage and recovery: Research and clinical perspectives.* New York: Academic Press, 1982.

Fromm, D. *Investigation of movement/EMG parameters in apraxia of speech.* Unpublished master's thesis, University of Wisconsin, Madison, 1981.

Goldstein, K. *Die transkortikalen Aphasien.* Fischer: Jena, 1915.

Grillner, S. Possible analogies in the control of innate motor acts and the production of speech. In S. Grillner, B. Lindblom, J. Lubker, & A. Persson (Eds.), *Speech Motor Control.* New York: Pergamon Press, 1982.

Hammarberg, R. On redefining coarticulation. *Journal of Phonetics,* 1982, *10,* 123-137.

Hardy, J. Lung function of athetoid and spastic quadriplegic children. *Developmental Medicine and Child Neurology,* 1964, *6,* 378-388.

Hardy, J. Suggestions for physiological research in dysarthria. *Cortex,* 1966, *3,* 128-156.

Hardy, J. Development of neuromuscular systems underlying speech production. In *Speech and the dentofacial complex: The state of the art.* 1970, *ASHA Reports,* (No. 5), 49-68.

Harris, F. Control of gamma efferents through the reticular activating system. *American Journal of Occupational Therapy*, 1969, *23*, 397-409.

Harris, F. Inapproprioception: a possible sensory basis for athetoid movements. *Journal of the American Physical Therapy Association*, 1971, *51*, 1971.

Hunker, C., Abbs, J., & Barlow, S. The relationship between parkinsonian rigidity and hypokinesia in the orofacial system: A quantitative analysis. *Neurology*, 1982, *32*, 755-761.

Jankovic, J., & Patel, C. Brainstem origin of blepharospasm. *Neurology*, 1983, *33* Suppl 2, 162.

Johnston, M., & Coyle, J. Development of central neurotransmitter systems. In *The fetus and independent life* (Ciba Foundation Symposium 86), London: Pitman, 1981.

Jurgens, U. Neural control of vocalization in nonhuman primates. In H. Steklis & M. Raleigh (Eds.), *Neurobiology of social communication in primates*. New York: Academic Press, 1979.

Kent, R. Cinefluorographic studies of dysarthria (Research Grant NS11022). Bethesda, MD: National Institutes of Health, 1973.

Kent, R. Articulatory-acoustic perspectives on speech development. In R. Stark (Ed.), *Language behavior in infancy and early childhood*. New York: Elsevier/North-Holland, 1981.

Kent, R. Brain mechanisms of speech and language with special reference to emotional interactions. In R. Naremore (Ed.), *Language Science*. San Diego: College-Hill Press, 1984.

Lenneberg, E. *Biological foundations of language*. New York: Wiley Press, 1967.

Lenneberg, E. The effect of age on the outcome of central nervous system disease in children. In R. Isaacson (Ed.), *The neuropsychology of development*. New York: Wiley & Sons, 1968.

Lhermitte, F., Derouesne, J., & LeCours, A. Contribution to the study of semantic disorders in aphasia. *Rev. Neurol.*, 1971, *125*, 81-101.

Linebaugh, C., Baird J., Baird, C., & Armour, R. Special considerations for the development of microcomputer-based augmentative communication systems. In W. Berry (Ed.), *Clinical Dysarthria*. San Diego: College-Hill Press, 1983.

Logemann, J., Fisher, H., Boshes, B., & Blonsky, E. Frequency and co-occurrence of vocal tract dysfunction in the speech of a large sample of Parkinson patients. *Journal of Speech and Hearing Disorders*, 1978, *43*, 47-57.

Lubker, J. Spatio-temporal goals: Maturational and cross-linguistic variables. In S. Grillner, B. Lindblom, J. Lubker, & A. Persson (Eds.), *Speech motor control*. New York: Pergamon Press, 1982.

Luria, A. *Traumatic aphasia*. Mouton: The Hague, 1970.

Luria, A. *Language and cognition*. New York: Wiley & Sons, 1981.

MacLean, P. The triune brain, emotion and scientific bias. In F. Schmitt (Ed.), *The Neurosciences: Second study program*. New York: Rockefeller University Press, 1970.

MacNeilage, P. Personal communication, 1983.

McCusker, E., Rudick, R., Honch, G., & Griggs, R. Recovery from the locked-in syndrome. *Archives of Neurology*, 1982, *39*, 145-147.

Meader, C., & Muyskens, J. *Handbook of biolinguistics, part 1: The structures and processes of expression.* Baltimore: Waverly Press, 1950.

Moore, J. Neuroanatomical considerations relating to recovery of function following brain injury. In P. Bach-y-Rita (Ed.), *Recovery of function: Theoretical considerations for brain injury rehabilitation.* Baltimore: University Park Press, 1980.

Morris, S. *Pre-Speech Assessment Scale: A Rating Scale for the Measurement of Pre-Speech Behaviors from Birth Through Two Years.* Milwaukee: Cerebral Palsy Project-Curative Rehabilitation Center, 1980.

Mountcastle, V. An organizing principle for cerebral function: The unit module and the distributed system. In G. Edleman & V. Mountcastle (Eds.), *The mindful brain.* Cambridge, MA: MIT Press, 1978.

Muller, E., Abbs, J., & Kennedy, J. Some systems physiology considerations for vocal control. In M. Hirano & K. Stevens (Eds.), *Vocal fold physiology.* Tokyo: University of Tokyo Press, 1981.

Muyskens, J. *The hypha.* Doctoral dissertation, University of Michigan, Ann Arbor, 1925.

Mysak, E. *Pathologies of speech systems.* Baltimore: Williams & Wilkins, 1976.

Mysak, E. *Neurospeech therapy for the cerebral palsied: A neuroevolutional approach.* New York: Teachers College Press, 1980.

Netsell, R. Physiological bases of dysarthria (Research Grant NS09627). Bethesda: National Institutes of Health, 1971.

Netsell, R. The acquisition of speech motor control: A perspective with directions for research. In R. Stark (Ed.), *Language behavior in infancy and early childhood.* New York: Elsevier/North-Holland, 1981.

Netsell, R. Speech motor control and selected neurologic disorders. In S. Grillner, B. Lindblom, J. Lubker, & A. Persson (Eds.), *Speech motor control.* New York: Pergamon press, 1982.

Netsell, R. Speech motor control: Theoretical issues with clinical impact. In W. Berry (Ed.), *Clinical dysarthria.* San Diego: College-Hill Press, 1983.

Netsell, R. & Daniel, B. Dysarthria in adults: Physiologic approach to rehabilitation. *Archives of Physical Medicine and Rehabilitation,* 1979, *60,* 502-508.

Oller, D. Infant vocalizations: Exploration and reflexivity. In R. Stark (Ed.), *Language behavior in infancy and early childhood.* New York: Elsevier/North-Holland, 1981.

Penfield, W., & Roberts, L. *Speech and brain mechanisms.* Princeton, NJ: University Press, 1959.

Perkell, J., & Nelson, W. Articulatory targets and speech motor control: A study of vowel production. In S. Grillner, B. Lindblom, J. Lubker, & A. Persson (Eds.), *Speech motor control.* New York: Pergamon Press, 1982.

Peterson, G., & Shoup, J. A physiologic theory of phonetics. *Journal of Speech Hearing Research,* 1966, *9,* 5-6.

Platt, L., Andrews, G., Young, M., & Neilson, P. The measurement of speech impairment of adults with cerebral palsy. *Folia Phoniatrica,* 1978, *30,* 50-58.

Ploog, D. Phonation, emotion, cognition, with reference to the brain mechanisms involved. *Ciba Foundation Symposium,* 1979, *69,* 78-98.

Ploog, D. On the neural control of mammalian vocalization. *Trends in Neuroscience,* 1981, *4,* 135-137.

Prechtl, H. Fargel, J., Weinmann, H., & Bakker, H. Postures, motility and respiration of low-risk pre-term infants. *Developmental Medicine and Child Neurology,* 1979, *21,* 3-27.

Pribram, K. Brain mechanism in music: Prolegomena for a theory of meaning. In M. Clynes (Ed.), *Music, mind, and brain: The neuropsychology of music.* New York: Plenum Press, pp. 21-35, 1982.

Rieber, R. *Language development and aphasia in children.* New York: Academic Press, 1980.

Robinson, I. *The new grammarians' funeral: A critique of Noam Chomsky's linguistics.* New York: Cambridge University Press, 1975.

Rosenbek, J., & LaPointe, L. The dysarthrias: Description, diagnosis, and treatment. In D.F. Johns (Ed.), *Clinical management of communicative disorders.* Boston: Little, Brown, 1978.

Rosenberg, R. Clinical neurochemistry. Shortcourse presented to the 35th Meeting of the American Academy of Neurology, San Diego, 1983.

Rubow, R. Biofeedback and the treatment of speech disorders. Biofeedback Society of America, 1980.

Rubow, R., Rosenbek, J., Collins, M., & Celesia, G. Reduction of hemifacial spasm and dysarthria following EMG feedback. *Journal of Speech Hearing Disorders,* in press.

Rutherford, D. Auditory-motor learning and the acquisition of speech. *Amer. J. Phys. Med.* 1967, *46,* 245-251.

Shohara, H. *Genesis of articulatory movements in speech.* Doctoral dissertation University of Michigan, Ann Arbor, 1932.

Shohara, H. Significance of overlapping movements in speech. *Proceedings of the Second Biennial Central Zone Conference of the American Society for the Hard of Hearing,* 1939.

Stetson, R. *Motor phonetics.* Amsterdam: North-Holland, 1950.

Tinbergen, N. On the aims and methods of ethology. *Zeit. t. Tierpsychol.* 1963, 410-433.

Vogel, M., & Cramon, D. von. Dysphonia after traumatic midbrain damage: A follow-up study. *Folia Phoniatrica,* 1982, *34,* 150-159.

Wall, P.D. Mechanisms of plasticity of connection following damage in adult mammalian nervous systems. In P. Bach-y-Rita (Ed.), *Recovery of function: Theoretical considerations for brain injury rehabilitation.* Baltimore: University Park Press, 1980.

Warwick, R., & Williams, P. *Gray's anatomy.* Philadelphia: W.B. Saunders, 1973.

Weismer, G., & Cariski, D. On speakers' abilities to control speech mechanism output: theoretical and clinical implications. In N. Lass (Ed.), *Speech and language: Advances in basic research and practice* (Vol. 10). New York: Academic Press, in press.

Wolff, P. Theoretical issues in the development of motor skills. *Symposium on Developmental Disabilities in the Pre-School Child.* Chicago: Johnson & Johnson, 1979.

Wolff, P. Normal variation in human maturation. In K. Connolly & H. Prechtl (Eds.), *Maturation and development: Biological and psychological perspectives* Philadelphia: J.B. Lippincott, 1981.

Yorkston, K.M., & Beukelman, D.R. Ataxic dysarthria: Treatment sequences based on intelligibility and prosodic considerations. *Journal of Speech Hearing Disorders,* 1981, *46,* 398-404.

ACKNOWLEDGMENTS

Preparation of this manuscript was supported by the Boys Town National Institute and an NIH research grant (NS 16763). L. D'Antonio and J. Rosenbek made helpful editorial comments and C. Dugan provided her usual excellence in manuscript preparation.

2

Respiratory Kinematics in Speakers with Motor Neuron Disease

Anne H. B. Putnam
Thomas J. Hixon

INTRODUCTION

Motor neuron disease is a family of degenerative illnesses affecting motor nerve cells in the spinal cord and brain. Its expression in the human neuromuscular system may vary from a so-called "benign" form, which progresses slowly among lower motor neurons, to an acute form, amyotrophic lateral sclerosis (ALS), which progresses rapidly, ravaging upper as well as lower motor neurons (Brooke, 1977). When bulbar motor neurons innervating the laryngeal or upper airway musculature are involved (as in progressive bulbar palsy, or in ALS), a dysarthria with flaccid or spastic signs, or both, may result, the perceptual characteristics of which have been well documented (Darley, Aronson, & Brown, 1975; Dworkin, Aronson, & Mulder, 1980). When spinal motor neurons innervating the trunk musculature are involved (as in progressive spinal muscular atrophy, or in ALS), wasting and weakness of chest wall muscles (those of the rib cage, diaphragm, and abdomen) may result in deterioration of respiratory function. This chapter is concerned with the effects on respiratory behaviors of motor neuron disease in the spinal motor system.

Information about changes in respiratory function associated with motor neuron disease comes primarily from clinical observations of patients with the ALS form of the disease. Their respiratory status often declines rapidly and they usually succumb to respiratory complications (for example, atelectasis, aspiration pneumonia, or congestive heart failure) because of reduced ventilatory efficiency (Brooke, 1977; Fallat & Norris, 1980; Keltz, 1965; Kreitzer, Saunders, Tyler, & Ingram, 1978). Some observers of respiratory function in motor neuron disease have described a pattern of anterior horn cell degeneration which may compromise the diaphragm, or the abdomen, earlier or more extensively than the rib cage (Fromm, Wisdom, & Block, 1977; Miller, Mulder, Fowler, & Olsen, 1957; Nakano, Bass, Tyler, & Carmel, 1976; Parhad, Clark, Barron, & Staunton, 1978). This focal pattern of deterioration has implications for respiratory function in general and perhaps also for respiratory support for speech. Heretofore, however, the effects of motor neuron disease on respiration for speech have not been studied systematically.

Existing clinical information on the respiratory capabilities for speech in individuals with motor neuron disease is primarily inferential, deduced from data for nonspeech respiration tasks and from patients' reports. Unfortunately, respiratory signs of dysarthria characteristic of motor neuron disease are rarely evaluated by the neurologist or the speech–language pathologist. The respiratory apparatus is crucial to sound production in the laryngeal and upper airways, and apparent disorders of voice and articulation in patients with motor neuron disease may be related to a disorder of respiration. Furthermore, the compensatory tolerance of the respiratory apparatus to the ravages of motor neuron disease may be different from that of the larynx and upper airway articulators with respect to the threshold for overt signs of disorder vis-'a-vis the demands of speech. Thus, whether or not the respiratory apparatus is involved, and if so, to what extent, constitutes information essential to the accurate evaluation and appropriate management of dysarthria presented by individuals with motor neuron disease.

This chapter summarizes a 3-year investigation of respiratory behavior in a group of adult subjects with motor neuron disease. It was our purpose to document the effects of their disease, if any were discernible, on the behavior of the chest wall,specifically with respect to the demands of speech. We studied respiratory function during speech in these subjects by means of the chest wall kinematic analysis procedure of Hixon, Goldman, and Mead (1973). We chose this procedure because of its investigative and clinical utility. It is noninvasive, risk free, can be applied efficiently and systematically to a large group of subjects, and requires no performance sophistication on the part of those to whom it is applied. Furthermore, there are reliable data on normal chest wall behaviors available in the literature (Hixon et al., 1973), as well as data on chest wall behaviors in disordered populations, including speakers with profound hearing impairment (Forner & Hixon, 1977), neuromuscular disorders (Hixon, 1982; Putnam, Hixon, & Stern, 1982; Hixon, Putnam, & Sharp, 1983), and voice disorders related to functional misuse of the respiratory apparatus (Hixon & Putnam, 1983).

METHOD

Subjects

Subjects of this investigation were 10 adult males with motor neuron disease. Their ages ranged from 34 to 72 years, and their histories of motor neuron disease from 3 to 12 years. Pertinent information on members of the group is presented in Table 2-1, including perceptual judgments of six aspects of their speech. In every case, the neuromuscular disorder had been diagnosed on the basis of health history, neurological examination, and electrodiagnostic studies; and, in many cases, a limb muscle biopsy had been taken. All of the subjects had at least spinal motor neuron involvement (MNDsp) with noticeable wasting and weakness in their limb and trunk musculature. All were ambulatory, though some required the assistance of canes or walkers. Most complained of mild to severe orthopnea, the subjective sensation of breathing difficulty when supine. Three of the subjects also had bulbar motor neuron involvement (MNDb) with signs or symptoms of laryngeal (CW), velopharnyngeal (FM and FG), labial (FM and FG), or lingual muscle weakness (FM, FG, and CW), and a noticeable dysarthria. Four of the subjects, including the three with bulbar signs, also exhibited upper motor neuron signs and carried the diagnosis of ALS.

Measurement Theory

The theoretical and technical details of chest wall kinematic analysis can be found elsewhere (Hixon et al., 1973; Hixon, Mead, & Goldman, 1976; Konno & Mead, 1967; Mead, Peterson, Grimby, & Mead, 1967). We shall review briefly those aspects of the theory which are germane to this investigation at this juncture and as the need arises later in the text. In kinematic theory, the chest wall is considered a two-part system consisting of the rib cage and diaphragm–abdomen[1] arranged in mechanical parallel. The chest wall surrounds the pulmonary system, which consists of the lungs and lower airways. The rib cage and abdomen each displace volume as they move, and their combined volume displacement equals that of the lungs. Changes in the anteroposterior diameters of the rib cage and abdomen have been shown to be linearly related to the volume each displaces. Therefore, the volume displaced by the rib cage and ab-

TABLE 2-1

Information on the subjects of this investigation pertinent to their physical characteristics, extents and histories of motor neuron disease, and the perceived disorder of their speech.

Subject	Age (yr)	Height (cm)	Diagnosis/Years	Voice Quality	Articulation	Nasal Resonance	Breath Group Duration	Utterance Loudness	Utterance Rate
EC	65	183	MNDsp/6	normal	normal	normal	normal	normal	normal
RF	34	169	MNDsp/3	strained-strangled*	normal	normal	short**	normal	normal
RR	46	178	MNDsp/5	normal	normal	normal	normal	normal	normal
KG	41	185	MNDsp/12	slightly tremorous	normal	normal	normal	normal	normal
VB	61	168	MNDsp/5	normal	normal	normal	normal	normal	normal
FM	72	165	MNDsp-b/8 (ALS)	strained-strangled	imprecise	hypernasal***	short	loud	slow
LC	66	179	MNDsp/?	normal	normal	normal	normal	normal	normal
FG	61	173	MNDsp-b/5 (ALS)	strained-strangled	imprecise	hypernasal***	short	loud	slow
KS	49	178	MNDsp/10 (ALS)	normal	normal	normal	normal	normal	normal
CW	68	170	MNDsp-b/3 (ALS)	strained-strangled*	normal	normal	short	normal	normal

*Calculated laryngeal airway resistance was abnormally high (Smitheran & Hixon, 1981).

**This subject exhibited a consistently laconic communication pattern in conversation; breath group duration in reading was normal.

***Concomitant aeromechanical coupling was verified instrumentally via nasal air flow measurements (Thompson & Hixon, 1979).

domen can be estimated from their respective diameter changes. An efficient method for measuring chest wall part diameter changes uses magnetometer coils attached to surface points of the rib cage and abdomen (Hixon et al., 1973). Typically, two generator–sensor coil pairs are used. The components of one pair are attached to the midline of the rib cage, front and back; the components of the other pair are comparably placed on the abdomen. These coils are elements in two electromagnetic transduction systems; each pair converts a chest wall part diameter change into a voltage analog which can be adjusted electronically and interpreted for volume displacement information.

The derivation of displacement information from diameter changes of the chest wall is predicated on the principle that each chest wall part moves with a single degree of freedom. That is, each part can assume only one shape at any given volume of that part. It is necessary, however, to calibrate the relationship between the anteroposterior diameter change of each part and its associated volume displacement. This calibration can be established conveniently by means of a chest wall adjustment called an isovolume maneuver, which is performed by the subject with the magnetometers in place. This maneuver reveals the functional relationships between the relative motion of the rib cage and abdomen at particular lung volumes, and allows for on-line conversion of the magnetometric signals from diameter change information to volume displacement information. The use of isovolume maneuvers in this investigation is described further in the Procedure section.

Instrumentation

The instrumentation for kinematic measurement and analysis in this investigation is schematized in Figure 2-1. As described above, magnetometers were used to sense the anteroposterior diameter changes of the rib cage and abdomen; their signals were displayed on-line oscilloscopically and stored simultaneously on two channels of an FM tape recorder for subsequent playback. The speech of the subject and commentary of the investigators were transduced by a microphone and recorded on a third channel of the FM tape recorder.

Procedure

The magnetometers were attached to the subjects' chest walls with double-sided adhesive tape. As shown in Figure 2-1, generating coils were positioned at the midline on the anterior surface of the chest wall, one for the rib cage near the level of the nipples, and one for the abdomen just above the navel. Sensing coils were positioned posteriorly on the midline at the same torso levels as their generator mates.

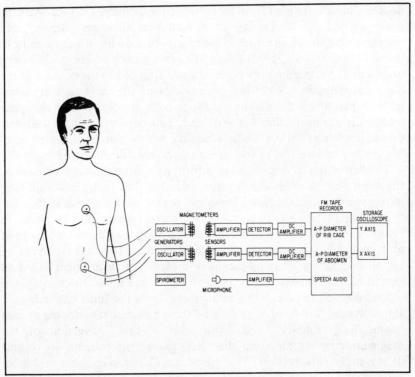

FIGURE 2-1
Schematic illustration of the instrumentation used for kinematic measurement and analysis in this investigation. See text for explanation.

The performance demands of the investigation were designed to optimize data collection without overtaxing the subjects' emotional or physical endurance. Accordingly, the protocol included only those nonspeech respiratory tasks necessary to calibrate and otherwise define kinematic landmarks unique to each subject's chest wall, several speech or speechlike tasks which simulated everyday communication demands, and multiple opportunities for resting tidal respiration. As illustrated in Figure 2-2, subjects performed these tasks in two body positions: first while seated upright,[2] and then while lying supine on a foam pad with a small pillow for head support. Five subjects with severe symptoms of orthopnea were not included in the supine position data collection. Subjects were instructed to avoid as much as possible raising their arms or shifting their body positions during the procedure.

The nonspeech respiration tasks included vital capacity maneuvers, resting tidal respiration, and isovolume maneuvers. Three vital capacity maneuvers were performed by each subject, and an average vital capacity

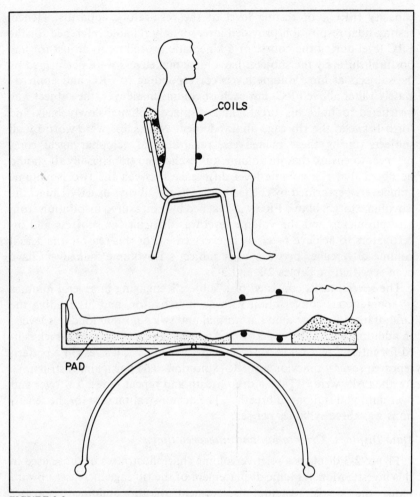

FIGURE 2-2
Schematic illustration of the body positions (seated upright and supine) in which subjects
performed the tasks of this investigation.

was computed and compared to the subject's predicted vital capacity
(using the formula weighted for age and height suggested by Comroe,
Foster, Dubois, Briscoe, & Carlsen, 1962). A 9-liter respirometer was
used to obtain the vital capacity data, and each subject wore a nose clip
during his performance of these maneuvers to preclude any loss of
volume transnasally. Data for approximately 30 sec of resting tidal
respiration were obtained between every task in the protocol. The tidal
end-expiratory level usually corresponds to the functional residual

capacity (FRC), or resting level of the respiratory appartus. Hence, resting tidal respiration provided a reasonably reliable reference for the FRC level during the course of a kinematic procedure to adjust for any postural shifts by the subject. Isovolume maneuvers were performed by the subjects at lung volume levels corresponding to FRC and approximately 1 liter above FRC. For each isovolume maneuver, the subject was instructed to hold his breath and displace volume slowly back and forth between the rib cage and abdomen. Nose clips were worn by all subjects during these maneuvers, regardless of velopharyngeal competence, to ensure that no volume was exchanged transnasally. It should be noted that the volume level difference between the two isovolume maneuvers performed by each subject was not always exactly 1 liter; the isovolume target above FRC was reached by a measured inspiration from a respirometer, and the volume level was difficult for subjects and investigators to achieve precisely in every case. For this reason, the actual volume differences between each subject's isovolume maneuvers have been specified in Tables 2-2 and 2-3.

The speech tasks consisted of a subject's engaging in several minutes of spontaneous conversation with an investigator, and his reading the Grandfather Passage aloud at normal and twice-normal loudness levels. In addition, each subject performed a syllable repetition task, which called for intermittent rapid, discrete increments in vocal stress in a pattern repeated several times on a single expiration. The particular instructions for the tasks were, "Take a deep breath and repeat /ta ta 'ta/ over and over until you run out of breath." The demonstration rate for the repetitions was three syllables per sec.

Data Displays: Orientation and Interpretation

Figure 2-3 displays a relative volume chart illustrative of those used in this investigation. Volume displacement of the rib cage increases upward along the *y*-axis; volume displacement of the abdomen increases rightward along the *x*-axis; and their combined volume displacement (that is, that of the lungs) increases upward along the diagonal axis. The solid diagonal lines in Figure 2-3 are isovolume lines. Each represents the relative volume pathway followed as volume is shifted back and forth slowly between the rib cage and abdomen with the airway closed at a fixed lung volume level. The two lines shown represent the FRC level and a level 1 liter above FRC. It is the isovolume maneuver and the isovolume pathway thus derived which facilitates conversion of diameter change information transduced by the magnetometer coils into relative volume displacements. That is, during the isovolume maneuver, the volume exchanged between the two chest wall parts is equal and opposite, provided

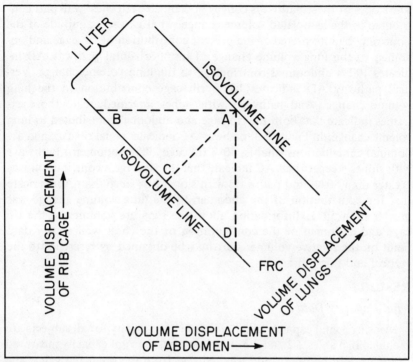

FIGURE 2-3
Relative volume chart (rib cage versus abdomen) illustrative of those used in this investigation. See text for explanation.

the airway is closed. Thus, to make the data on the chart read as if equal volume changes occurred for equal diameter changes of the rib cage and abdomen, the magnitudes of the coil signals are adjusted electronically during the performance of an isovolume maneuver so that the line representing the volume shift on the chart has a slope of − 1.

Relative to the axes and the isovolume lines on a relative volume chart, any series of data points forming a pathway graphs the changing shape of the chest wall during a respiratory behavior such as a tidal respiration cycle or a single expiratory breath group in speech. These pathways can be interpreted to reveal lung volume changes, relative contributions of the rib cage and abdomen to such volume changes, the separate volumes of the rib cage and abdomen, and the configuration of the chest wall. For example, the concomitant change in lung volume along a kinematic pathway can be estimated from the distance between any two points perpendicular to the isovolume lines (Hixon et al., 1973). Thus, pathways AB, AC, and AD in Figure 2-3 each chart 1-liter changes in lung volume.

The slopes of these pathways convey how much each chest wall part contributed to the associated volume change. That is, the magnitude of the slope may be interpreted as the percent contribution of rib cage and abdomen to the lung volume change. Thus, horizontal pathway AB indicates 100% abdominal contribution to the lung volume change. Vertical pathway AD indicates 100% rib cage contribution to the lung volume change. And pathways with slopes intermediate to those extremes indicate that both the rib cage and abdomen contributed to lung volume change. In Figure 2-3, pathway AC indicates equal rib cage and abdominal contributions (that is, 50% rib cage, 50% abdomen). Pathways with slopes steeper than AC indicate that the rib cage's contribution was greater than 50%, and pathways with slopes less steep than AC indicate that the contribution of the abdomen to the lung volume change was greater than 50%. Information about the separate volumes of the rib cage and abdomen or the configuration of the chest wall at any data point on the relative volume chart may be obtained by reference to the vertical and horizontal axes.

RESULTS

Vital Capacity Data

Measured vital capacity and predicted vital capacity for all subjects are included in Tables 2-2 and 2-3. In every case, the vital capacity measured in the upright body position was reduced from the predicted value; the measured values ranged from 39 to 98% of predicted. For those five subjects from whom supine position data were obtained, measured vital capacities were slightly larger than, comparable to, or smaller than those obtained from the same subjects upright; the capacity change in the supine position ranged from 3% higher to 52% lower than comparable upright values.

Resting Tidal Respiration — Upright

Upright resting tidal volumes (in liters, L), frequencies (in breaths per minute, BPM), minute volume rates (in liters per minutes, LPM), and percentages of rib cage and abdominal contributions to lung volume change are listed in Table 2-2 for all subjects in the upright body position. Resting tidal volumes ranged from 0.25 to 1.00 L; frequencies ranged from 13 to 25 BPM, and minute volume rates from 4.75 to 15 LPM. Characteristic resting tidal respiration patterns of volume displacement are illustrated in Figures 2-4a and 2-4b. The pathways shown in the figures represent both inspiration and expiration. The slopes of the resting tidal respiration pathways on the charts reflect that both the rib cage and the abdomen contributed to volume displacement, though the

TABLE 2-2
Numerical data for respiratory tasks in the upright body position.

| | Vital Capacity | | | | Resting Tidal Respiration | | |
Subject	Measured (L)	% Predicted	Volume (L)	Frequency (BPM)	Minute Volume (LPM)	% Contribution RC/AB	Isovolume Line Difference (L)
EC	2.40	65*	0.60	25	15.00	57/43	1.20
RF	3.46	87	0.45	19	8.55	71/29	1.15
RR	2.68	67*	0.60	16	9.60	41/59	1.00
KG	4.18	98	1.00	13	13.00	89/11	1.20
VB	3.16	91	0.65	14	9.00	91/9	1.05
FM	2.90	90	0.75	13	9.75	56/44	1.00
LC	3.47	96	0.70	14	9.80	90/10	1.10
FG	1.40	39*	0.25	19	4.75	56/44	1.00
KS	2.30	59*	0.30	22	6.60	33/67	1.00
CW	2.23	66*	0.45	25	11.25	90/10	1.00

*Indicates abnormally reduced from predicted.

TABLE 2-3
Numerical data for respiratory tasks in the supine body position.

Subject	Vital Capacity			Resting Tidal Respiration			
	Measured (L)	% Differs from Upright	Volume (L)	Frequency (BPM)	Minute Volume (LPM)	%Contribution RC/AB	Isovolume Line Difference (L)
FM	2.90	0	0.70	17	11.90	30/70	1.15
KS	2.37	3>	0.40	22	8.80	48/52	1.00
KG	3.30	9<	0.90	8	7.20	25/75	1.05
VB	3.22	2>	0.70	13	9.10	39/61	1.05
CW	1.15	52<	0.35	24	8.40	61/39	0.85

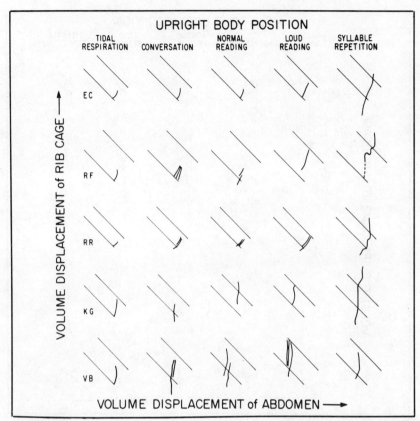

FIGURE 2-4a
Relative volume charts for subjects EC, RF, RR, KG, and VB in the upright body position showing representative data for resting tidal respiration, conversation, normal reading, loud reading, and syllable repetition tasks. The long diagonal lines (-1 slopes) are isovolume pathways, the lower one at FRC and the upper one approximately 1 liter above FRC. See Table 2-2 for precise isovolume line separation in each subject's charts. Data pathways include the remaining solid and dashed lines on the subjects' charts.

contribution of the rib cage tended to predominate in most cases. Note that the pathway slopes are not constant, however. The predominant contribution of the rib cage increased (that is, the slopes steepen) at the higher volume ends of the quiet respiration cycles for most of the subjects. Estimates of the percent of rib cage and abdominal contribution to lung volume change in these data were made from the most extensive portion of each pathway exhibiting a relatively constant slope. Based on this measurement scheme, rib cage contribution to lung volume displacement during upright resting tidal respiration was estimated to range from

50   *The Dysarthrias*

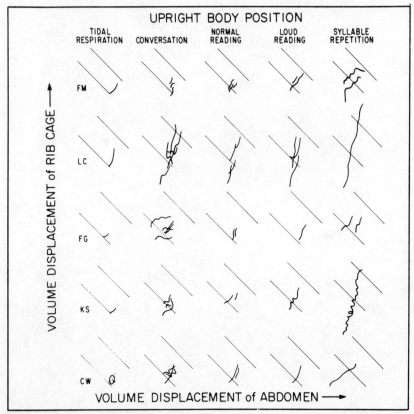

FIGURE 2-4b
Relative volume charts for subjects FM, LC, FG, KS, and CW in the upright body position
showing representative data for resting tidal respiration, conversation, normal reading,
loud reading, and syllable repetition tasks. The long diagonal lines (minus one slopes) are
isovolume pathways, the lower one at FRC and the upper one approximately 1 liter above
FRC. See Table 2-2 for precise isovolume line separation in each subject's charts. Data
pathways include the remaining solid and dashed lines on the subjects' charts.

33 to 91%, and abdominal contribution from 9 to 67%. One conspicuous pathway deserves individual comment here, the looped configuration in the tidal respiration data of subject CW (Figure 2-4b). After
his first few tidal breaths (dashed pathway), his tidal pathway began to
loop clockwise. The left side of the loop on his chart represents tidal inspiration, and the right side with the arrowhead, tidal expiration.

Resting Tidal Respiration — Supine

Supine tidal volumes, frequencies, minute volume rates, and relative
contributions of the rib cage and abdomen to lung volume change are

listed in Table 2-3 for the five subjects from whom data were collected in this body position. Supine resting tidal volumes ranged from 0.35 to 0.90 L; frequencies ranged from 8 to 24 BPM, and minute volume rates from 7.2 to 11.9 LPM. The volume displacement patterns for supine resting tidal respiration are displayed in Figure 2-5. Conspicuous in these data are the looped pathways on all the subjects' charts; both inspiratory and expiratory volumes are represented,with arrowheads marking expiration. The loops cycle counterclockwise in four of the subjects, and clockwise in the fifth, CW. Relative volume slopes were roughly estimated as the long axis of each ellipse. Based on this measurement scheme the rib cage contribution to supine resting tidal volume exchange ranged from 25 to 61%, and the abdominal contribution from 39 to 75%.

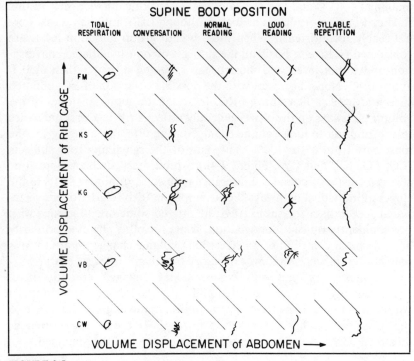

FIGURE 2-5
Relative volume charts for subjects FM, KS, KG, VB, and CW in the supine body position showing representative data for resting tidal respiration, conversation, normal reading, loud reading, and syllable repetition tasks. The long diagonal lines (−1 slopes) are isovolume pathways, the lower one at FRC and the upper one approximately 1 liter above FRC. See Table 2-3 for precise isovolume line separation in each subject's charts. Data pathways include the remaining solid lines on the subjects' charts.

Conversation — Upright

Data for the subjects' conversational speech in the upright position are illustrated in Figures 2-4a and 2-4b. Each pathway represents a single expiratory breath (that is, one linguistic breath group). Often a cluster of such pathways are shown to illustrate breath group pattern variation across a series of consecutive utterances. In other cases, subjects were so consistent in their patterns that a single pathway represents chest wall displacement seemingly regardless of linguistic load or length of utterance differences across breath groups. The lung volume levels at which subjects initiated conversation differed. Four subjects (KG, VB, FM, and KS) tended to initiate conversation at or below their resting tidal end-inspiratory levels, four (EC, RF, RR, and CW) tended to begin at levels slightly higher than their tidal end-inspiratory levels, and the remaining two (LC and FG) typically began speaking at twice their resting tidal end-inspiratory levels or higher (though LC's initiation levels were noticeably inconsistent). When these breath group initiation levels are considered relative to FRC, all the subjects obviously initiated conversation above that level, and most began speaking at better than 0.50 L above FRC. None, however, with the possible exception of LC, initiated speech at levels a liter above FRC. In six of the subjects, slopes of the volume pathways on the charts generally reflect a rib cage predominance in contribution to lung volume change during utterance, ranging for the most part from 65 to 100%. The data of the remaining four subjects (LC, FG, KS, and CW, Figure 2-4b) exhibit marked changes in slope across a cluster of connected utterance pathways, or abrupt shifts in the slopes of individual pathways. For example, note the cluster of conversational speech data for subject FG; he uttered some breath groups with predominantly rib cage contribution, while for others he used primarily an abdominal contribution to effect lung volume change. Subject CW's data cluster indicates that his expiratory breath groups were characterized frequently by pathways whose slopes changed abruptly from predominantly rib cage to predominantly abdominal contributions within the same breath group. Furthermore, in the unusual slope data of these four subjects and perhaps even a fifth (FM), the pathways often indicate paradoxical displacements of the rib cage and the abdomen.[3]

Conversation — Supine

The data for conversation in the supine body position are illustrated in Figure 2-5. The lung volume levels at which subjects initiated conversation differed. Starting levels ranged from approximately the tidal end-inspiratory level to approximately twice the tidal volume depth. Relative to the FRC of each subject, the supine conversation initiation levels of three (KG, VB, and FM) were often a liter or more above FRC, though VB began at that level only rarely, and FM showed a noticeable decrease in starting level over time. The remaining two subjects (KS and CW) never initiated supine conversation a liter above FRC. The slopes of the data pathways changed abruptly in all but one of the supine subjects, FM, in whom the rib cage contribution to lung volume displacement was 60%. Among the other four supine subjects, the abruptly changing slopes, with some evidence of rib cage and abdominal paradoxing, had been noted already in the upright conversational data of two, KS and CW, but were novel for KG and VB.

Reading — Upright

The displacement data for the subjects' readings of the Grandfather Passage in the upright body position at normal and twice-normal loudness levels are illustrated in Figures 2-4a and 2-4b. Six of the subjects (EC, RF, RR, VB, FM, and LC) tended to initiate normal reading near or below their resting tidal end-inspiratory levels, three (FG, KS, and CW) began at levels somewhat higher than their tidal end-inspiratory levels, and one (KG) initiated his reading considerably higher than his tidal end-inspiratory volume. Considering these initiation levels relative to FRC, nine subjects typically initiated normally-loud upright reading at volumes less than a liter above FRC. Only KG initiated his reading a liter or more above that level. When instructed to read the passage at twice-normal loudness, seven of the subjects initiated utterances at lung volume levels higher than their normal reading starting levels. Two subjects (CW and LC) exhibited essentially no change in lung volume initiation levels between the two reading conditions, and one subject (KG) initiated loud reading at lower lung volume levels than those at which he had read the passage normally. The slopes of the pathways in all cases indicate that both chest wall parts contributed to lung volume displacement during the reading tasks, though in general, the rib cage tended to predominate more or less. There are examples, however, of pathways where equal contributions of rib cage and abdomen to lung volume change are apparent (see, for example, RR or FM), or where the contribution is exclusively that of the rib cage (see VB). Subject KS exhibited some abrupt changes in the pathway slopes of his breath groups during the loud reading performance with chest wall part paradoxing similar to that which characterized his conversational data.

Reading — Supine

The data generated by the supine subjects for reading are illustrated in Figure 2-5. Lung volume initiation levels for normally-loud reading were roughly comparable to or below resting tidal end-inspiratory levels in one subject (KG), and somewhat higher in the other four (FM, KS, VB, and CW). Among the latter, however, only VB initiated his reading a liter or more above FRC, though inconsistently so. Four subjects' attempts at loud reading were usually initiated higher than the lung volume levels at which they had begun reading normally; subject KG, however, tended to initiate the loud reading at or below his normal reading initiation level. Slopes of the pathways for reading supine in three subjects (KG, VB, and CW) exhibited a number of abrupt shifts in chest wall part contribution to lung volume displacement with evidence of rib cage and abdominal paradoxing within a single expiratory breath group, though CW was inconsistent with respect to this characteristic between the two reading conditions. Subjects FM and KS exhibited data slopes without numerous abrupt shifts in either reading condition, though their data in the loud reading performance do exhibit several gradual changes in slope.

Syllable Stress Task — Upright

Data generated by the subjects on the syllable repetition stress task in the upright body position are illustrated in Figures 2-4a and 2-4b. In six cases (EC, RF, RR, KG, LC, and KS) subjects initiated this task at lung volume levels at least a liter or more above FRC (in response to the instruction, "Take a deep breath"). Five of these six also continued the task below FRC (as per instructions to continue "until you run out of breath"). The sixth subject, RF, always stopped performing the task well above FRC, however, and expired quietly to FRC as indicated by the dashed portion of his relative volume pathway for this activity (Figure 2-4a). The remaining four subjects generated data which were initiated at much lower levels. Two of these (VB and FG) also produced data which were curtailed at end-task level, stopping at or just below FRC; the other two (FM and CW), though they started at low lung volumes, were able to continue the task well below FRC. The slopes of the pathways generated by the subjects on this task exhibit several patterns. Four subjects (EC, KG, VB, and LC) generated data in which a rib cage contribution to lung volume change prevailed. Other subjects (RF, RR, FM, FG, and KS) exhibited slopes in which the predominance of rib cage and abdomen alternated abruptly in contribution to lung volume change. In the cases of FM and KS, the abrupt shifts in the pathways were consistently related to the occurrence of stressed syllables during utterance of the task; in the other cases, such shifts in chest wall part contributions were apparently unrelated to the occurrence of stressed syllables. There are numerous signs of rib cage or abdominal paradoxing in the data; the signs are subtle in subjects RR, KG, and VB, and obvious in RF, KS, and CW whose pathway reflects noticeable abdominal paradoxing as he began the task and then equal contributions of rib cage and abdomen to lung volume displacement as he continued. There are also indications of rib cage paradoxing among the abrupt slope changes in the data of RF and FM.

Syllable Stress Task — Supine

The data generated by the supine subjects for this task are illustrated in Figure 2-5. Lung volume initiation levels were more than a liter above FRC in two subjects (FM and KS), and less than a liter above FRC in the other three. At the termination level of the task, FM, VB, and CW ended at FRC; KS and KG continued below FRC. The slopes of the displacement pathways for four subjects (KS, KG, VB, and CW) exhibit abrupt shifts in chest wall part contributions to lung volume change consistently related to the occurrence of stressed syllables in the task. In addition, there is more or less evidence of paradoxical motion of the abdomen among the abrupt slope changes for those four subjects and an occasional sign of rib cage paradoxing. The data of FM show slight changes in slope, which were apparently unrelated to the occurrence of stressed syllables during utterance, with evidence of abdominal paradoxing near the end of one performance.

DISCUSSION

It is of interest first to discuss the data for vital capacity maneuvers and resting tidal respiration. These provide some insight into the basic ventilatory capabilities of the subjects on which demands for speech were superimposed. Measured vital capacities for all subjects in the upright body position were reduced from predicted values. A measured vital capacity is not considered abnormally low, however, unless it is reduced by more than 20% of the predicted value (Comroe et al., 1962). Applying this criterion to the measured upright vital capacity data of our subjects, the values of five were within normal limits of variation. The values of the remaining five (asterisked in Table 2-2) were markedly reduced, ranging from 39 to 67% of predicted. When body position is shifted from upright to supine, a small change in the measured vital capacity, usually a reduction, is not unexpected (Comroe et al., 1962). Hence, for four of our subjects, supine vital capacity values varied slightly from upright in unremarkable amounts. Subject CW, however, exhibited a

52% reduction in vital capacity when shifted from upright to supine. What information do such remarkable differences convey with respect to the effect of motor neuron disease on the respiratory apparatus?

Reduction in the measured upright vital capacity from expected values has been cited often as a consequence of neuromuscular disease when the chest wall musculature is involved (Comroe et al., 1962; Gibson, Pride, Newsom Davis, & Loh, 1977; Kreitzer et al., 1978; McCredie, Lovejoy, & Kaltreider, 1962; Nakano et al., 1976; Newsom Davis, Stagg, Loh, & Casson, 1976b; Stone & Keltz, 1963). The discrepancy between measured and predicted vital capacity may be attributed to fatigue, weakness, or both, in any one or all of the chest wall components. A large discrepancy between the vital capacity measured in the upright and supine positions, with the latter remarkably reduced, has been associated with diaphragmatic weakness. In the supine position, gravitational forces normally effect an inward displacement of the abdominal wall and a headward displacement of the diaphragm which, when relaxed, may encroach on the expiratory reserve volume and alter the mechanical constraints,on the chest wall. Such constraints as well as an increase in pulmonary blood volume in this position (Comroe et al., 1962), may render the supine measured vital capacity reduced slightly from upright values. If the diaphragm is weak or paralyzed, it may also be displaced headward passively during inspiration in the supine position, thus reducing the efficiency of the remaining inspiratory muscles. This imposes a limitation on the inspiratory capacity and may greatly exaggerate a normal tendency toward a reduced vital capacity when supine. This phenomenon may explain the 52% reduction in measured vital capacity for subject CW when he was shifted from upright to supine. His data resemble those reported by McCredie et al. (1962) and Newsom Davis, Goldman, Loh, and Casson (1976a) on patients with documented diaphragm paresis or paralysis who tended to exhibit supine vital capacities reduced by 50% or more from their upright values.

Consider the resting tidal respiration data. Compared to the normal resting tidal volume range of 0.45 to 0.60L (Comroe et al., 1962), four of our subjects had upright resting volumes within normal limits, two fell below, and four fell above the normal range. In the supine postion, one subject fell below, one within, and three above the normal limits. Compared to the normal resting tidal frequency range of 11 to 14 BPM (Comroe et al., 1962), four of our upright subjects fell within the average normal range, and six had abnormally high resting tidal frequencies. In the supine position, one subject fell below, one within, and three above the normal frequency range. When the resting tidal depths and frequencies are considered in terms of minute volume rates, the normal reference is 5.2

to 8.8 LPM (using normative data of Comroe et al. (1962), applied to the nomogram of Radford, Ferris, & Kriete (1954), and corrected for altitude). Relative to these figures, in the upright position one of the subjects fell below that range, two fell within it, and seven exceeded it. In the supine position, three of the subjects fell within the normal range, and two exceeded it.

Alterations in the depth and frequency of resting tidal respiration and changes in minute volume rates have a well-documented association with weakness of the respiratory muscles. Small resting tidal volumes and rapid tidal frequencies, such as those seen in six of our subjects upright and three supine, have been cited as characteristic of chest wall weakness, especially diaphragmatic, and accompanied by laboratory evidence of hypoventilation (Newson Davis et al., 1976a,1976b; Gibson et al., 1977; Fromm et al., 1977; Parhad et al., 1978) and decreased diffusing capacity (Nakano et al., 1976). High resting minute volume rates, such as those seen in seven of our subjects upright and two supine, have been associated with unnecessary alveolar hyperventilation in patients with restricted chest wall excursion due to respiratory muscle weakness in motor neuron disease (Kreitzer et al., 1978) or secondary to spinal cord trauma (Stone & Keltz, 1963), and resemble respiratory behaviors induced experimentally by chest wall strapping in normal subjects (Gibson et al., 1977). In this context it is also appropriate to comment on the implications of orthopnea which was reported as a more-or-less troublesome symptom by most of our subjects. Orthopnea is the subjective sensation of breathing difficulty when supine, with or without accompanying evidence of ventilation–perfusion abnormality. It is acknowledged as a symptom in many patients with neuromuscular disorder of the chest wall and may be suggestive of weakness or fatigue in any or all of the chest wall parts. Because the symptom characterizes supine respiration, however, flaccid paresis or paralysis of the diaphragm, or spastic paresis or paralysis of the abdominal wall, or both, are most often implicated due to an exaggeration of the normal effects of the supine position on the mechanical behaviors of these two chest wall components when they are disabled by neuromuscular disorder (Miller et al., 1957; Comroe et al., 1962; McCredie et al., 1962; Stone & Keltz, 1963; Newsom Davis et al., 1976a; Parhad et al., 1978).

Thus far, given their tendency toward reduced vital capacities and systematic alterations in the temporal and volumetric characteristics of resting tidal respiration, accompanied by frequent reports of orthopnea, our subjects' data are consistent with a picture of chest wall muscle weakness — particularly inspiratory — presented in the literature on disordered respiration in neuromuscular disease. With the preceding information in mind, consider the relative volume data for resting tidal respiration. In general, the slopes of the pathways reflect normal patterns of chest wall part contributions to volume displacement, the contribution of the rib cage predominating in most of the subjects upright, and the contribution of the abdomen predominating in most of the supine subjects (Hixon et al., 1973). These normal tendencies notwithstanding, there are two unusual details in the specific configuration of the tidal respiration pathways which deserve discussion. Normal relative displacement patterns for quiet respiration usually form a single, relatively straight pathway for both inspiration and expiration (Hixon et al., 1973). Many of the quiet respiration data of our subjects, however, exhibited unusual hooked or looped configurations. For example, most of the upright resting tidal pathways are noticeably hooked toward the y-axis at their higher volume ends where the slopes of the pathways become remarkably steeper. This unusual configuration denotes a shift to more rib cage contribution near the end of inspiration, with evidence of abdominal paradoxing in RF and VB, perhaps reflecting fatigue of the diaphragm's contribution to the inspiratory gesture.

The other configuration among the data for resting tidal respiration which is unusual is a looped pathway which appears on the chart of subject CW in the upright position, and on the charts of all the supine subjects. CW, after his first few resting tidal breaths upright (which exhibited a hooked configuration; note the dashed line in Figure 2-4b), produced a pathway which looped in a clockwise direction. The inspiratory pathway which forms the left side of the loop denotes motion of the rib cage in the inspiratory direction but motion of the abdomen in the expiratory direction. Furthermore, it should be noted that CW's neck muscles bulged visibly during each inspiration. The expiratory path of his loop denotes rib cage displacement in the expiratory direction but abdominal displacement in the inspiratory direction. This relative volume pattern and associated neck muscle activity on inspiration were also characteristic of his resting tidal respiration when supine. If these kinematic data are coupled with his vital capacity and numerical tidal respiration statistics, the picture is consistent with signs of diaphragm weakness. Specifically, his abnormally reduced upright measured vital capacity (66% of predicted); the abnormally large reduction in his supine measured vital capacity compared to his upright value (down 52%); his low resting tidal volume, high tidal frequency, and high minute volume rate; kinematic pathways which imply paradoxing of the abdominal wall during portions of both inspiration and expiration (Newsom Davis et al., 1976a); and a habitual tendency to assist inspiration with neck muscle effort, all suggest that his diaphragm, normally a major muscle of inspiration, was not normally active during his resting tidal inspiration in either body position.

The other looped pathways in the resting tidal respiration data were characteristic of the supine data of four subjects and followed a counterclockwise course. The inspiratory sides of the loops follow the expected pattern for this body position (Hixon et al., 1973), but uncharacteristic of normal subjects, the expiratory pathways are displaced to the left of the inspiratory data. This leftward deviation implies that the subjects used expiratory muscular forces of the rib cage and the abdomen, and perhaps more predominantly the latter, to facilitate lung volume displacement for the duration of resting tidal expiration,which is normally a predominantly passive phenomenon involving relaxation forces during its last two-thirds (Hixon et al., 1973). Several explanations may be offered for this behavior. Since all four subjects complained of mild to moderate orthopnea, their tidal expiratory muscle efforts may represent a strategy to take some active control over a usually passive process and offset the emotional discomfort of orthopneic symptoms (McCredie et al., 1962). It is also conceivable that these tidal expiratory muscle gestures, whose slopes suggest considerable abdominal contribution, may be strategies to facilitate subsequent inspiration when the diaphragm is mildly weak and easily fatigued (Newsom Davis et al., 1976a). That is, abdominal muscle efforts during tidal expiration may ensure headward displacement of the diaphragm to a position which is mechanically advantageous for its next inspiratory contraction; and, relaxation of the abdominal muscles at the end of a tidal expiration may be helpful in initiating footward motion of the diaphragm during the subsequent inspiration (though this latter strategy would be more effective with the torso upright, the position for which it was reported by Newsom Davis et al., 1976a and Gibson et al., 1977).

Consider now the kinematic data for conversation and reading. The placement of these data on the relative volume charts provides information about the background torso configuration prevailing during the chest wall displacement charted. Our reference point for placement was the intersection of a subject's resting tidal expiratory pathway with his FRC isovolume line.[4] In Figures 2-4a and 2-4b, note that the data for conversing and reading upright tend to cluster on the charts slightly to the left of where each tidal expiration pathway intersected the FRC line. This is consistent with the normal torso configuration for speech upright in which the rib cage tends to be larger and the abdomen smaller than their presumed relaxed configurations at the prevailing lung volume. In Figure 2-5, the data for conversing and reading supine tend to cluster on the charts slightly to the right of the tidal end-expiration points. This, too, is consistent with normal chest wall shape for speech supine in which the rib cage is smaller and the abdomen larger than their presumed relaxed configurations at the prevailing lung volume. These data placements imply that our subjects had sufficient strength in their chest walls to assume a normal torso configuration for these speech activities.

Abnormalities in the data for conversation and reading include low lung volume initiation levels and abrupt changes in chest wall part contributions to lung volume displacement during utterance. Consider the lung volume initiation level discrepancy first. Normal talkers typically begin normally-loud utterance at about twice their resting tidal depths and, depending on the linguistic load and individual phrasing styles, typically end utterance at or just above FRC (Hixon et al., 1973). The majority of our 10 subjects, however, failed to initiate conversation or normally-loud reading at the expected lung volume level in either body position, and many initiated utterance no higher than their resting tidal end-inspiratory levels. For the loud reading, most of the subjects demonstrated that they were able to initiate speech at higher lung volume levels than those at which they had read normally, as normal speakers are wont to do for loud utterance (Hixon et al., 1973). That they did so only when compelled, however, and often lapsed in their efforts before the reading passage ended, suggests that the more forceful inspirations necessary for the load reading were effortful maneuvers which they could not perform repetitively without fatigue or discomfort. These data are consistent with the suggestion of inspiratory muscle weakness noted in other respiratory performances of these subjects.

Low lung volume levels of speech initiation can be a liability to utterance length and to the expiratory recoil they provide for utterance loudness. Furthermore, when inspiratory muscle weakness is coupled with significant expiratory muscle weakness, low levels of initiation may compromise both volume displacement and volume compression in the expiratory direction. The weak expiratory muscles of the rib cage are not stretched to an optimal mechanical advantage, and the abdomen may be a weak opposing partner to rib cage compression. This may translate to inadequate loudness for sound generation and stress contrasts as well as short breath groups in speech, not to mention ineffectual power for more strenuous chest wall activities like coughing and clearing secretions (Brooke, 1977; Kreitzer et al., 1978; Fallat & Norris, 1980). Among these possible consequences of low lung volume initiation levels in speech, only short breath groups were a noticeable sign in three of our subjects (CW, FM, and FG) at the time of this investigation. Among these three, only CW's short phrases could be attributed exclusively to chest wall weakness. (He had high laryngeal airway resistances [Smitheran & Hix-

on, 1981] and no perceptible signs of upper airway valving incompetence.) Subjects FM and FG, however, in addition to exhibiting
signs of respiratory weakness, also demonstrated pervasive
velopharyngeal incompetence during speech, forfeiting much of their expiratory flow transnasally. In their cases, both respiratory and upper airway inadequacies probably combined to reduce the pressure and flow
available for speech production on any one expiration.

Before leaving this issue of the implications and liabilities of low lung
volume initiation levels in speech, one other aspect deserves consideration in the interest of patient management and counseling. When the
kinematic data reveal signs of inspiratory muscle weakness, it would be
helpful to know the extent to which the weakness is partitioned between
the rib cage and diaphragm. In this investigation, only the data of CW
provide enough nonspeech and speech information to support specific
implication of the diaphragm as the weak inspiratory component. The
apparently reduced inspiratory capabilities of many of the other subjects, though suggestive, are not so readily attributable to either inspiratory rib cage or diaphragm weakness without further information.
To resolve this ambiguity, and a similar one which could arise for expiration between the rib cage and abdomen, investigators and clinicians
would do well to assess the inspiratory and expiratory reserve volumes in
subjects with motor neuron disease and to monitor the kinematics of
their chest walls during tasks which compel their use of these extremes of
the vital capacity.

The other abnormality of interest in the data for conversation and
reading among our subjects was the appearance of unusual changes in
slope along the volume displacement pathways. Comparable data for the
normal chest wall manifest slope changes during utterance,though such
changes tend to be gradual. Furthermore, when normal slopes change in
steepness during utterance, their direction is still more-or-less downward
and leftward on the relative volume chart indicating in-phase motion of
the rib cage and abdomen in the expiratory direction (Hixon et al., 1973).
The slope data of some of our subjects were aberrant for both these
characteristics. First, the slope changes were noticeably abrupt and frequent within a single breath group, indicating numerous seemingly erratic changes in chest wall part contributions to lung volume
displacement. And second, the direction of some of the pathways after
an abrupt change in slope often coursed upward and leftward on the
charts indicating paradoxical motion of the rib cage, or downward and
rightward indicating paradoxical motion of the abdomen. Four subjects
exhibited these erratic pathways during conversational speech in the
upright position. However, none of these, or any others, exhibited such

aberrations when reading at normal loudness levels upright. In the supine position, all but one of the five subjects demonstrated the unusual pathway changes in conversation, and three of the five also demonstrated them in reading at both loudness levels. Considering the performance contexts in which the aberrant slope data were observed, note that they were more or less apparent depending on the constraints of the material uttered and the body position in which the speech behavior was elicited. Yet they were not associated with any perceptible changes in utterance quality or loudness. What, then, could be the significance of these unusual but acoustically unobtrusive behaviors of the chest wall?

Pertinent to the interpretation of these data is the fact that the chest wall affected by motor neuron disease undergoes considerable neuromuscular reorganization (Brooke, 1977). Hence, the speaker with motor neuron disease must adjust his respiratory pump for speech with a neuromuscular system whose control properties are altered and perhaps even deficient as a result of motor neuron death, chest wall muscle atrophy, and susceptibility to fatigue. Under these circumstances, the kinematic evidence of abrupt exchanges between chest wall parts for predominance in lung volume displacement during utterance may represent rib cage/abdominal "groping" as a consequence of reduced afferent feedback for fine motor control of chest wall part coordination due to loss of proprioceptors in atrophied muscle. It is also conceivable that the "trade-off" between efforts of the rib cage and abdomen during utterance may be strategies to counteract fatigue in their respective muscle groups, which has been well-documented as a troublesome symptom and noticeable sign in muscles affected by motor neuron disease (Norris, Denys, & Ü, 1980).

That the unusual slope data were more or less apparent depending on tasks and body position may also be interpreted in terms of disordered chest wall control capabilities. In the upright body position, the unusual slopes characterized the kinematic data of some subjects' conversation but not their reading. The utterance constraints imposed by the reading task may have given the subjects finite expiratory phrasing boundaries within which to organize speech breathing support strategies. Consecutive conversational utterances, on the other hand, were spontaneous and had to be grouped into expiratory gestures extemporaneously by the subjects. Of these two speech tasks then, reading and spontaneous consecutive conversation, the unrehearsed or unmarked nature of the latter might be more likely to challenge fine motor control of the chest wall for on-line adjustments. In the supine position, the aberrant slopes were apparent not only in the conversational speech data of four of the five subjects, but also in the reading data of three of the five. Furthermore, for two of these, the unusual pathway shifts during utterance were novel characteristics not having been apparent in their upright data. That these unusual slope changes were more prevalent in the supine position may imply that the relatively unrehearsed nature of speech supine challenges fine motor control of the disordered chest wall even more than speech behaviors upright. It is also conceivable that the respiratory load of speaking while lying supine might exaggerate a subject's orthopnea, and his anxiety (McCredie et al., 1962),while speaking under such conditions might be reflected in the erratic interplays between the rib cage and abdomen. Whatever their explanation, these unusual slope data and the variation in their prevalence with speech mode and body position may have important implications for the identification and management of a respiratory disorder in motor neuron disease and deserve further investigation.

Finally, this discussion would not be complete without some consideration of the syllable-repetition-with-alternating-stress tasks. These showed variation across subjects with respect to lung volume initiation and termination levels and unusual patterns of chest wall part contributions to lung volume change, including evidence of rib cage and abdominal paradoxing. Nevertheless, all the subjects met the task demands of the stress pattern /tɑ tɑ ˈtɑ/. Hence, to the extent that a talker uses the chest wall as a major contributor to the loudness increase associated with heavy stress on every third syllable of the utterance pattern, all our subjects were able to muster the muscle forces necessary to imitate the stress pattern requested.[5] It is difficult to interpret the kinematic data for this task in relation to chest wall weakness. For example, the number of times a subject could repeat a triad on one breath varied from one to as many as 15 times and appeared to be associated with the depth of inspiration that preceded the task as well as the lung volume at which the subject chose to terminate the task. But, such level differences could be attributed to things other than neuromuscular weakness. Subjects differed in their interpretations of the instructions as well as their abilities to follow them, even with a model to imitate. Some were admittedly inhibited about performing such a nonsense task in the presence of their spouse and strangers. Others appeared to be unwilling to push their respiratory apparatuses to inspiratory or expiratory extremes to comply with the instructions. And, we use "unwilling" here not in a pejorative way but simply to convey that the weakness and fatiguability which characterize muscular systems affected by motor neuron disease exert emotional as well as physical limitations on subjects' abilities to use these systems, regardless of their intents to be cooperative.

CONCLUSIONS

The numerical vital capacity and tidal respiration data obtained from the subjects of this study were aberrant in ways suggestive of chest wall muscle weakness, particularly in the inspiratory direction, and consistent with pulmonary function data on similar groups of subjects in the literature. The chest wall kinematic data complemented the numerical data with information about chest wall displacement during tidal respiration and speech, which also suggests inspiratory muscle weakness and possibly some disorder of chest wall coordination during utterance. It is important to consider these data in practical relation to the respiratory demands of everyday speech and the expected destruction pattern of motor neuron disease. Normal speakers in the upright body position produce conversation between 60 and 40% of the vital capacity (40 and 20% supine); this amounts to approximately 20% of the average adult male 5-liter vital capacity (Hixon et al., 1973). Thus, conversational speech normally demands and consumes only a moderate portion of the midrange lung volume. An extensive literature on respiratory function for nonspeech tasks in subjects with motor neuron disease, some of which had been referred to here, reports that chest wall muscle weakness and wasting, whether generalized or focal, tends first to curtail the inspiratory and expiratory extremes of the lung volume range. Thus, one might reasonably expect that such weakness would have to be extensive in all parts of the chest wall, or selectively and profoundly destructive to one of the chest wall components to encroach noticeably on the midvolume range of the vital capacity and compromise respiration for conversational speech. Based on our study of these 10 subjects who differed extensively in age, history, and distribution of signs and symptoms of motor neuron disease, that expectation appears to be a valid one. To be sure, some subjects exhibited unusual patterns of chest wall part contribution to lung volume displacement during speech, and most subjects initiated speech tasks at low lung volume levels. All, however, were still able to muster adequate volume displacement and, apparently, volume compression for the demands of conversation, in spite of the kinematic signs of chest wall muscle weakness or disordered control. Unfortunately, such signs, though subtle in most of the subjects at the time of this investigation proved to be liabilities to their pulmonary health and harbingers of further neuromuscular deterioration.

NOTES

[1]The diaphragm-abdomen behaves mechanically as a single structure. Its inner surface is the diaphragm, its outer the abdominal wall, and its incompressible center the abdominal contents (Hixon et al., 1973). Hereinafter, the diaphragm–abdomen will be referred to as "abdomen", though diaphragm–abdomen is always implied.

[2]Note that upright body position data were obtained while subjects were seated, rather than standing, which is the standard reference position (Hixon et al., 1973). The subjects could not tolerate standing and maintaining a stable posture for the one-half hour required to complete the procedure in the upright position. Instead, they were seated in a straight-backed chair with their torsos stabilized (but unrestrained) in an upright position they could maintain consistently during the procedure. Shifting from standing to sitting upright may effect a small reduction in the vital capacity (2%) due to changes in the effects of gravity on the chest wall and encroachments on the rib cage volume by headward displacement of the abdominal contents (Campbell, Agostoni, & Newsom Davis, 1970). These changes are small, however, and one would not predict that substantially different data patterns would be generated with the subjects seated instead of standing. As a control measure, however, we obtained seated upright data from a group of neuromuscularly normal men who matched the subjects with motor neuron disease on the basis of age and height. On perusal of the control group's data, we were satisfied that for the respiratory activities of interest, the relative volume patterns of the normal subjects seated upright were consistent with data for normals standing upright.

[3]Paradoxical displacements of the rib cage or abdomen are ones in which the displacement of the part is opposite in sign to lung volume displacement.

[4]The reference points for assessing appropriate placement for kinematic data on relative volume charts traditionally have been the *relaxed* configurations of the chest wall at the prevailing lung volumes (Hixon et al., 1973; Hixon et al., 1976). The relaxation maneuvers required to establish such reference points are tedious, however, and were not included in our protocol. Instead, we chose to use the tidal end-expiratory level as a reference: It usually corresponds to the resting level (FRC) of the respiratory apparatus, and the point at which the tidal expiratory pathway intersects the FRC isovolume line most nearly approaches the relaxed configuration of the chest wall at that level.

[5]We noted that our subjects also tended to make the stressed syllables higher in frequency and longer in duration, which are two other parameters which can be manipulated to create the perceptual impression of heavy stress.

REFERENCES

Brooke, M. *A clinician's view of neuromuscular diseases.* Baltimore: Williams & Wilkins, 1977.

Campbell, E., Agostoni, E., & Newsom Davis, J. *The respiratory muscles: Mechanics and neural control.* Philadelphia: Saunders, 1970.

Comroe, J., Forster, R., Dubois, A., Briscoe, W., & Carlsen, E. *The lung: Clinical physiology and pulmonary function tests.* Chicago: Year Book Medical Publishers, 1962. 2nd ed.

Darley, F., Aronson, A., & Brown, J. *Motor speech disorders.* Philadelphia: Saunders, 1975.

Dworkin, J., Aronson, A., & Mulder, D. Tongue force in normals and dysarthric patients with amyotrophic lateral sclerosis. *Journal of Speech and Hearing Research,* 1980, *23,* 828–837.

Fallat, R., & Norris, F. Respiratory problems. In D. Mulder (Ed.), *The diagnosis and treatment of amyotrophic lateral sclerosis.* Boston: Houghton-Mifflin, 1980.

Forner, L., & Hixon, T. Respiratory kinematics in profoundly hearing-impaired speakers. *Journal of Speech and Hearing Research,* 1977, *20,* 373–408.

Fromm, G., Wisdom, P., & Block, A. Amyotrophic lateral sclerosis presenting with respiratory failure. *Chest,* 1977, *71,* 612–614.

Gibson, G., Pride, N., Newsom Davis, J., & Loh, L. Pulmonary mechanics in patients with respiratory muscle weakness. *American Review of Respiratory Disease,* 1977, *115,* 389–395.

Hixon, T. Speech breathing kinematics and mechanism inferences therefrom. In S. Grillner, B. Lindblom, J. Lubker, & A. Persson (Eds.), *Speech motor control.* New York: Pergamon Press, 1982.

Hixon, T., Goldman, M., & Mead, J. Kinematics of the chest wall during speech production: Volume displacements of the rib cage, abdomen, and lung. *Journal of Speech and Hearing Research,* 1973, *16,* 78–115.

Hixon, T., Mead, J., & Goldman, M. Dynamics of the chest wall during speech production: Function of the thorax, rib cage, diaphragm, and abdomen. *Journal of Speech and Hearing Research,* 1976, *19,* 297–356.

Hixon, T., Putnam, A., & Sharp, J. Speech production with flaccid paralysis of the rib cage, diaphragm, and abdomen. *Journal of Speech and Hearing Disorders,* 1983, *48.*

Hixon, T., & Putnam, A. Voice disorders in relation to respiratory kinematics. *Seminars in Speech, Language and Hearing,* 1983, *4,* 217–231.

Keltz, H. The effect of respiratory muscle dysfunction on pulmonary function. *American Review of Respiratory Disease,* 1965, *91,* 934–938.

Konno, K., & Mead, J. Measurement of the separate volume changes of rib cage and abdomen during breathing. *Journal of Applied Physiology.* 1967, *22,* 407–422.

Kreitzer, S., Saunders, N., Tyler, H., & Ingram, R. Respiratory muscle function in amyotrophic lateral sclerosis. *American Review of Respiratory Disease,* 1978, *117,* 437–447.

McCredie, M., Lovejoy, F., & Kaltreider, N. Pulmonary function in diaphragmatic paralysis. *Thorax,* 1962, *17,* 213–217.

Mead, J., Peterson, N., Grimby, G., & Mead, J. Pulmonary ventilation measured from body surface movements. *Science,* 1967, *156,* 1383–1384.

Miller, R., Mulder, D., Fowler, W., & Olsen, A. Exertional dyspnea: A primary complaint in unusual cases of progressive muscular atrophy and amyotrophic lateral sclerosis. *Annals of Internal Medicine,* 1957, *46,* 119–125.

Nakano, K., Bass, H., Tyler, H., & Carmel, R. Amyotrophic lateral sclerosis: A study of pulmonary function. *Disorders of the Nervous System,* 1976, *37,* 32–35.

Newsom Davis, J., Goldman, M., Loh, L., & Casson, M. Diaphragm function and alveolar hypoventilation. *Quarterly Journal of Medicine,* 1976, *45,* 87–100. (a)

Newsom Davis, J., Stagg., Loh, L., & Casson, M. The effects of respiratory muscle weakness on some features of the breathing pattern. *Clinical Science and Molecular Medicine,* 1976, *50,* 10p–11p. (b)

Norris, F., Denys, E., & Ü,K. Differential diagnosis of adult motor neuron diseases. In D. Mulder (Ed.), *The diagnosis and treatment of amyotrophic lateral sclerosis.* Boston: Houghton-Mifflin, 1980.

Parhad, I., Clark, A., Barron, K., & Staunton, S. Diaphragmatic paralysis in motor neuron disease. *Neurology,* 1978, *28,* 18–22.

Putnam, A., Hixon, T., & Stern, L. *Speech breathing function in Friedreich's ataxia.* Paper presented at the 19th annual meeting of the Federation of Western Societies of Neurological Science, San Diego, 1982.

Radford, E., Ferris, B., & Kriete, B. Clinical use of a nomogram to estimate proper ventilation during artificial respiration. *The New England Journal of Medicine,* 1954, *251,* 877–884.

Smitheran, J., & Hixon, T. A clinical method for estimating laryngeal airway resistance during vowel production. *Journal of Speech and Hearing Disorders,* 1981, *46,* 138–146.

Stone, D., & Keltz, H. The effect of respiratory muscle dysfunction on pulmonary function. *American Review of Respiratory Disease,* 1963, *88,* 621–629.

Thompson, A., & Hixon, T. Nasal air flow during normal speech production. *Cleft Palate Journal,* 1979, *16,* 412–420.

ACKNOWLEDGMENT

We gratefully acknowledge those who volunteered as subjects for this investigation. Also, for their interest in and cooperation with this research, we acknowledge Dr. Lawrence Z. Stern, neurologist, and the Muscular Dystrophy Association of Tucson, Arizona. This work was funded in part by grants from the National Institute of Neurological and Communciative Disorders and Stroke.

3

Physiological Analyses of Parkinsonian Tremors in the Orofacial System

Chauncey J. Hunker
James H. Abbs

INTRODUCTION

The large-scale effort of Darley, Aronson, and Brown (1969a, 1969b, 1975) offered a definitional framework on the multiple populations afflicted with motor speech disorders and thus a clear focal point for subsequent investigations. In summarizing that classical work, Darley et al. (1969a, 1969b) noted that their data should provide the basis for subsequent investigations into the physiological characteristics of dysarthria. Related to the expectations of Darley and his colleagues, efforts in clinical neurophysiology have begun to provide a quantitative basis for determining functional neuropathophysiology. Clinical neurophysiology, as pointed out by Stalberg and Young (1981), has flourished due to improved technology for studying the physiology of the human nervous system and its dysfunctions. The magnitude of this effort is reflected in the 10 volumes edited by J.E. Desmedt (1973-1982), in as many years, with contributions from more than 100 clinical and basic neuroscientists. Based on these substantial advances in research on the pathophysiology of movement disorders, some scientists in speech have embraced the goals of clinical neurophysiology in an attempt to bring new technical sophistication to the quantification of speech motor disorders. In this context, our particular efforts have been predicated on the expectation that quantitative, physiological assessment of motor speech disorders can, as in the area of clinical neurophysiology, "provide more concrete, fundamental information than offered by behavioral or linguistic approaches, and hence improve the foundation upon which to base programs of diagnosis, rehabilitation, or clinical research" (Abbs, Sutton, Larson, & Eilenberg, 1973). This chapter is thus a reflection of that focus.

The special relevance of and basic applied research in human instrumental neurophysiology for dysarthria is most apparent if one acknowledges that these disorders are fundamentally speech production system manifestations of a global neuromotor dysfunction. Thus, as with other movement disorders, the ultimate understanding for potential assessment and treatment must by definition be based on analyses of the associated aberrations in movement and muscle contraction. Without such analyses, motivated by specific hypotheses concerning underlying neural dysfunction, advances beyond surface classifications of global symptoms or new treatment techniques beyond "black box" trial and error are unlikely to be forthcoming.

Because of the relative newness of neurophysiological studies of motor speech disorders, the number of uncharted areas is beyond the scope of any given investigation, any single investigator, or even the most ambitious multifaceted descriptive project. Thus, this chapter will focus on a single neuromuscular symptom in a single dysarthric population; we will examine limb and orofacial motor data for the presence, nature, and underlying neural substrates of parkinsonian tremors. Incorporated into this chapter will be data from our own investigations, interpreted in relation to current hypotheses on the pathogenesis of tremors in Parkinson's disease and in terms of the relationship between these tremor forms and the concomitant movement aberrations. This focus may appear odd to many, given the classical clinical wisdom that tremor (1) may not be manifest in the orofacial system of parkinsonian dysarthrics and/or (2) is of little or no significance as a contributing factor to the associated speech motor impairments. However, in physiological observations of movement and muscle activity in the orofacial system of Parkinson subjects, we have commonly observed orofacial tremors of substantial magnitude (cf. Abbs, Hunker, & Barlow, 1983; Hunker, Abbs, & Barlow, 1982). Moreover, based on recent work in the limbs where engineering analysis techniques have been employed, it is apparent that tremor studies in the orofacial system may provide new indices with which to discern underlying neural pathway dysfunctions and to evaluate these aberrant mechanisms in relation to associated motor performance deficits (cf. Desmedt, 1978).

Tremor in the limbs has been characterized, according to Dejerine (1914) and most recently by Stein and Lee (1981), as involuntary, rhythmical oscillations superimposed on a fixed position or on a movement trajectory involving either the whole body or parts of it. Traditionally, different forms of pathological tremor have been distinguished by their association with the motor performance during which they occur (e.g., resting tremor, action tremor, and so on). In this regard, Struppler, Erbel, and Velho (1978) proposed a clinical classification of tremors by correlating them to four conditions of limb motor behavior: (1) optimal relaxation, (2) positioning against gravity, (3) volitional innervation (action), and (4) isolated goal-seeking movement (intention).

In addition to qualitative observations of limb tremor during various motoric conditions, efforts have been made to quantify the associated tremor frequencies by either calculating the time period of the basic oscillation, or more recently via spectral analysis. Several studies utilizing spectral analysis techniques have demonstrated that tremor is not a single regular oscillation as it may appear from oscillographic manifestations, but rather is a complex waveform composed of several different frequency components (Findley, Gresty, & Halmagyi, 1981; Freund & Dietz, 1978). Hence, based on the results of spectral analysis, it is not appropriate to consider pathological tremor as a periodic modulation of muscle activity at a single frequency. These results complicate the notion of tremor as a simple rhythmic process and require that a consideration of tremor mechanisms be undertaken with care. Further, based on instrumental monitoring and spectral analysis, it is apparent that many neurologically impaired populations, contrary to classical descriptions, manifest multiple forms of tremor as a function of the motor conditions observed. For example, in Parkinson's disease, using instrumental techniques, four forms of tremulous movements are evident in the limbs: resting tremor, postural tremor, action tremor, and cogwheeling. In subsequent sections of this chapter, we will (1) evaluate each of these forms of tremor, noting the conditions under which they are manifest in the limbs; (2) explore, using instrumental observations, the extent to which parallel tremor patterns are present in the speech production system; (3) offer some hypotheses concerning the performance impairments resulting from or correlated to these processes; and (4) indicate future directions for the use of tremor analyses in motor speech disorder assessment.

GENERAL METHODS

Because the tremors associated with Parkinson's disease are more varied than reflected in the classical literature, several parallel observations in any given subject (using different physiological measures) were necessary. For this reason, in this section, descriptions of methods will be confined to the subjects studied and the physiological measures employed. The motor performance conditions under which each major form of tremor was observed will be described in conjunction with the experimental results.

Subjects

Eight males with parkinsonian dysarthria were investigated in various portions of this study (cf. Table 3-1). While not all measures were obtained for all subjects, there was a sufficient degree of overlap to discern relevant trends. The subjects ranged in age from 37 to 77 years. All subjects were examined by a laboratory staff neurologist to ensure that they were free from secondary signs that are not typically associated with the classical Parkinson's disease profile. To avoid potential drug dosage-related response fluctuations, the experimental data were obtained only at the end of the anti-Parkinson medication dosage cycle. While these subjects varied in their drug treatment histories and the specific pharmacological agents in use, there was not a systematic relation between medications and the tremor profiles. This observation is consistent with Dietrichson, Engebretsen, Fonstelien, and Hovland (1978), who reported that while tremor amplitude fluctuated as a function of the particular anti-Parkinson medication in use, tremor frequency remained

TABLE 3-1
Age, duration of disease, and severity of dysarthria for each Parkinsonian patient

Subject	Age (yrs.)	Duration of disease (yrs.)	Severity of dysarthria
P1	77	10	Moderate
P2	72	22	Mild/moderate
P3	69	18	Moderate
P4	68	12	Mild/moderate
P5	64	19	Severe
P6	62	26	Severe
P7	62	7	Mild
P8	37	6	Mild/moderate

NOTE: The severity of the dysarthria was subjectively evaluated and agreed on by two clinical speech pathologists.

remarkably stable. Extensive observations from normal subjects ranging in age from 35 to 71 years were made for the same experimental conditions, and these data have been included for comparative purposes where it has been deemed necessary.

Physiological Measures

Movement. Upper lip, lower lip, and jaw movements were observed in the inferior-superior dimension using a headmounted strain gauge transduction system designed and constructed for this purpose (Barlow, Cole, & Abbs, 1983). This transduction system is ultra-lightweight and permits observation of these movements without fixing the subject's head. The bandwidth of each transducer (at least 40Hz) exceeds that of the lip movements for speech, and head movement artifact has been shown to be negligible (less than .5 mm).

Muscle activity. Activity of the perioral muscles were observed using hooked-wire, intramuscular electrodes consisting of 70-micron copper wire with enamel insulation; 2 mm of insulation were scraped from the recording tip. Each wire of a bipolar electrode pair was inserted with 30-gauge hypodermic needles with intraelectrode distances varying from 3 to 5 mm, depending on the size of the underlying muscle. These copper wire electrodes have been shown to have the bandwidth, noise floor, and resistance to movement artifact necessary for facial muscle recording during speech (Konopacki & Cole, 1982). EMG signals were amplified with a bandwidth of 50–2,500Hz. Electrode placement sites were based on previous anatomical studies (Kennedy & Abbs, 1979).

Isometric muscle force. Upper and lower lip isometric forces were transduced with specially designed transducers (Barlow & Abbs, in press). These transducers are sensitive in the force ranges required for speech of these individual articulators and have bandwidths adequate for observing human physiological tremors (greater than 100Hz).

Laryngeal vibrations. A Knowles (Model BU-1771) accelerometer was fixed on the skin overlying the thyroid lamina to transduce vibrations of the vocal folds. This transducer is not sensitive to airborne acoustic vibrations.

Speech acoustic waveform. In all tasks involving speech movements, the airborne speech waveform was transduced with a high quality dynamic microphone placed approximately 15 cm from the subject's lips.

These movement, force, EMG, and acoustic signals were transduced and recorded simultaneously on FM tape with a bandwidth of DC-2500

Hz for each channel. The particular signals analyzed varied with the experimental task. Signal analyses were implemented using a Hewlett-Packard 3582A real-time spectrum analyzer, a PDP-11/44 computer with special measurement/data summary algorithms, and/or hardcopy displays on a Honeywell optical oscillograph (1108) or a Tektronix 4662 digital plotter. All of the low frequency spectral measurements of the lip and jaw movement, force, and EMG data resulted from a root mean square averaging operation with a Hanning window on 20 task repetitions.

STUDY ONE: RESTING TREMOR

Brief rationale. Among the forms of aberrant oscillatory behavior, the classical resting tremor of the limbs is recognized as a clinically dominant feature of parkinsonism. Resting tremor frequently commences and remains most pronounced in the distal musculature of the upper extremities, where the combination of flexion-extension and pronation-supination gives rise to the characteristic "pill-rolling" oscillations. Resting tremor in the limbs is generally reported to occur at a major frequency within a range of 3.0 to 7.0Hz, with additional smaller amplitude oscillations that are harmonically related to the principle frequency (Findley et al., 1981; Stiles & Pozos, 1976; Wachs & Boshes, 1961). The tremor is rarely localized to one muscle group. Most often, the rhythmical activity is diffuse and involves all the muscles of an oscillating structure. Typical descriptions of the EMG recorded from antagonistic muscle groups during resting tremor indicate reciprocal, alternating bursts of activity occurring at 3.0 to 7.0Hz, synchronous with the tremor frequency. The amplitude of parkinsonian rest tremor is modulated by many factors. Although it is described as tremor of rest, complete relaxation and removal of sensory stimulation diminishes the amplitude of the tremor and it disappears completely during sleep. On the other hand, emotion, stress, and fatigue, as well as intellectual concentration, increase resting tremor amplitude (Growdon, Young, & Shahani, 1975; Rondot, Jedynak, & Ferrey, 1978). Because limb resting tremor has served traditionally as a distinguishing diagnostic symptom of parkinsonism, it is of particular interest to examine a possible orofacial system manifestation of this tremor in its classical form.

Specific tasks. To observe tremor at rest, the subjects were instructed to assume a facial resting position in which the lips were touching slightly and the facial, jaw, and laryngeal muscles were completely relaxed. Labial muscle activity was monitored throughout the experiment to ensure the absence of voluntary activation. The resting position was main-

tained for 20 intervals, with durations of 10 sec. each. Between resting intervals, subjects were asked to separate and moisten the lips and to

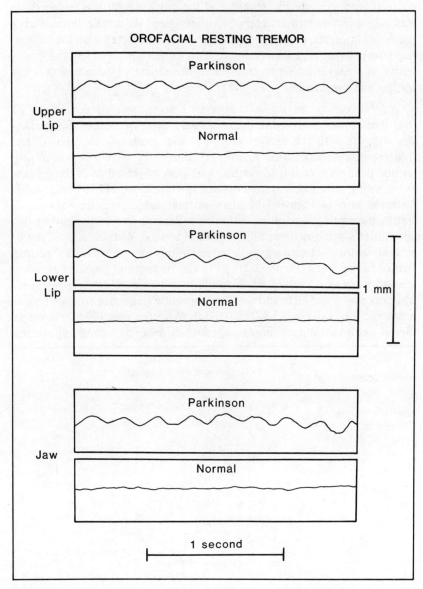

FIGURE 3-1
Oscillographic records obtained with the movement transduction system from the upper
lip, lower lip, and jaw positioned at rest from a Parkinsonian dysarthric and normal control
subject.

swallow; these maneuvers were to minimize tension and fatigue that could occur in maintaining the rest position. Under optimal conditions, subjects were completely relaxed and the environment was quiet; there was no subject-experimenter verbal interaction. At certain times during these rest intervals, the experimenter verbally interacted with the subject (e.g., to provide task instructions). This condition provided an opportunity to observe resting tremor when the subject's intellectual concentration was heightened.

Observations in the orofacial system. During optimal conditions of rest, tremor was observed in the orofacial system of each of the Parkinson subjects with the exception of P8, the youngest subject with the shortest disease duration. Figure 3-1 illustrates parkinsonian resting tremor in the upper lip, lower lip, and jaw, observed with the lip-jaw movement transduction system (as described in General Methods). As illustrated also in Figure 3-1, when normal subjects assume the same resting positions,the regular rhythmic oscillations seen in the parkinsonian subjects are not discernible. Spectral analysis of these signals reveal several features consistent with observations of parkinsonian resting tremor in the limbs (Figure 3-2). As in the fingers and limbs, the resting tremor in the orofacial system is complex, with a dominant resting spectral peak at 4.0 to 5.0Hz and smaller amplitude frequency components at harmonic intervals, (e.g., 8.0 to 9.0Hz). With the possible exception of the jaw, normal subjects show no spectral evidence of a dominant tremor

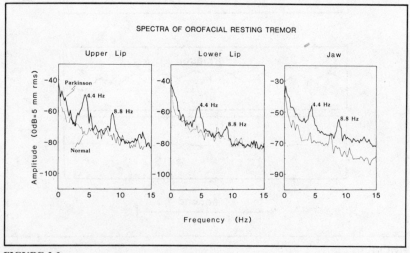

FIGURE 3-2
Comparison of the spectra from a normal (light line) and a Parkinson subject (dark line) for the upper lip, lower lip, and jaw during the resting condition.

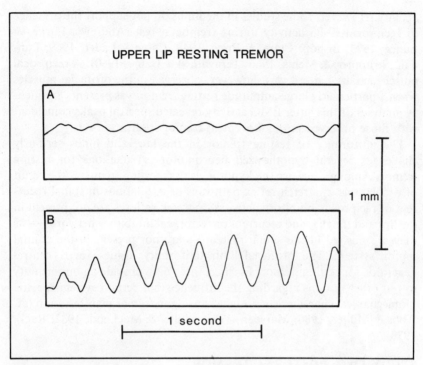

FIGURE 3-3
Comparison of the small amplitude (A) and large amplitude (B) resting tremor from one of the Parkinsonian dysarthrics.

peak. The parkinsonian tremor amplitudes were observed to fluctuate as a function of internal and external variables (i.e., intellectual concentration, fatigue, ambient noise). Figure 3-3 compares two samples of upper lip tremor obtained under different resting conditions from the same parkinsonian subject. The small amplitude tremor (Figure 3-3A) was transduced during a period of minimal environmental stimulation; the large amplitude sample (Figure 3-3B) was obtained a few seconds later while the experimenter presented task instructions. Comparable amplitude differences for these two conditions were noted in the upper lips, lower lips, and jaw for each Parkinson subject with resting tremor. These resting tremors were most frequently accompanied by asynchronous EMG activity in antagonist muscle pairs. Spectrally, the frequency composition of the EMG resembled "white noise" (i.e., a flat spectral response within the frequency range of interest). These findings are in contrast to most descriptions of resting tremor in the limbs and fingers which indicates rhythmic, reciprocal antagonistic muscle EMG activity. However, some studies in the limbs do not support the presence of reciprocal EMG activity during tremor at rest (Andrews, Burke, & Lance, 1973; Bishop, Clare, & Price, 1948; Calne & Lader, 1969; Landau, Struppler, & Mehls, 1966; Teravainen & Calne, 1980). A reciprocal muscle activity pattern was, however, observed in the orofacial muscles when a particularly large amplitude resting tremor was present. Frequency analyses of this latter EMG activity revealed spectral peaks coincident with those observed in the movement tremor spectra.

The uniformity of resting tremor in the face and limbs seriously challenges several hypothesized neuromotor explanations for resting tremor. Among these are the hypotheses that resting tremor is the result of oscillations of stretch reflex pathways or oscillations in spinal recurrent or reciprocal inhibitory networks. Stretch reflexes are not present in the lips and tongue, and recurrent or reciprocal inhibitory networks — as they are posited in the spinal system — are not present in the cranial motor system. The orofacial/limb uniformity argues for a central generator for resting tremor. Further, these data provide an opportunity to test other notions regarding the influence that certain system-specific biomechanical characteristics might have upon tremor manifestation (cf. Abbs & Müller, 1980; Marsden, 1978; Müller & MacLeod, 1982; Rack, 1978).

STUDY TWO: POSTURAL TREMOR

Brief rationale. According to the categorization proposed by Struppler et al. (1978), postural tremor occurs when the limbs or hands are maintained in an unsupported position against gravity in the absence of dynamic voluntary action. Stiles and Pozos (1976) described postural tremor in the hands of Parkinson patients as large amplitude oscillations which varied from 4.0 to 9.0Hz. This fluctuation in frequency was inversely related to the amplitude of the tremor. Findley et al. (1981) observed a postural hand tremor with a dominant spectral peak between 6.0 and 6.2Hz accompanied frequently by an additional, less dominant peak at 4.0 to 5.0Hz.

Freund and Dietz (1978) contend that spectral analysis of limb tremor under isometric force conditions (as a special postural condition) is a facile neurophysiological technique for discerning neuronal activities in a given tremor-generating muscle. The interpretation of these signals is more direct than frequency measurements obtained during resting or action tremor where many muscles differentially contribute to structural oscillations; during isometric conditions oscillations can be examined in a more controlled manner.

The spectral analyses of isometric forces recorded from the limbs and digits developed in an attempt to find a neurophysiologically valid method for discerning the activity of a motoneuron pool noninvasively; i.e., without having to record from single motor units. The validity of such an assessment has been verified by simultaneous analysis of single motor unit activity and muscle force tremor in the fingers and limbs of normal human and animal subjects and in various pathological subjects, including some with Parkinson's disease (Allum, Dietz, & Freund, 1978; Dietz, Bischofberger, Wita, & Freund, 1976; Dietz, Freund, & Allum, 1975; Dietz, Hillesheimer, & Freund, 1974; Elble & Randall, 1976; Freund, Budingen, & Dietz, 1975; Freund, Dietz, Wita, & Kapp, 1973; Milner-Brown, Fisher, & Weiner, 1979; Milner-Brown, Stein, & Yemm, 1973). These studies have shown that certain motor unit discharge characteristics (firing rate thresholds, firing rate modulation, and abnormal synchronization) are reflected in the muscle force spectral envelope (Freund & Dietz, 1978). More specifically, the low frequency range of the isometric force spectrum is produced by slow force variations due to changes in the net activity of the motoneuron pool. The high frequency range, including the dominant spectral peak, is produced by the unfused parts of the twitch contractions of all motor units firing at rates between recruitment and total fusion (cf. Figure 5 in Freund & Dietz, 1978). Hence, as proposed, the spectral analysis of force tremor provides a semiquantitative assessment of the range of firing rates over which the motoneuron pool operates under certain conditions and an indication of the proportion of units discharging at the various rates.

Freund (1982) most recently has proposed further that the peak frequency in the spectrum of isometric force, in addition to reflecting the motor unit firing rate thresholds, correlates highly with the fastest rate at which voluntary movements or muscle contraction can be executed. That is, when a subject is instructed to perform a maximally rapid alternating movement of finger or hand, the speed at which this movement is produced approximates the dominant frequency of the involuntary force tremor. Because the components of the speech production system dynamically assume various conditions of rest, posture, and movement differentially during speech production, it is of significance to examine the orofacial system output for tremor manifestations at neutral postures as well as during various levels of isometric contraction.

Specific tasks. Orofacial postural tremor was measured with the lips parted and the jaw lowered (i.e., a position comparable to the production of the vowel /ɑ/). Additional measures of postural tremor were obtained during controlled isometric (static) labial muscle contractions. For this latter task, the subject was instructed to match a target force level presented on an oscilloscope by compressing the lips against a bilabial force transducer. Each isometric contraction was sustained for 20 sec.

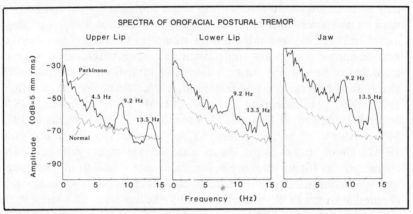

FIGURE 3-4
Comparison of spectra from a normal (light line) and a Parkinson subject (dark line) for the upper lip, and jaw during the postural condition.

Observations in the orofacial system. The postural tremor observed in the orofacial structures differed in spectral composition from that reported in the limbs and hands. Figure 3-4 illustrates representative spectral plots of postural tremor from the upper lip, lower lip, and jaw from Parkinson subject (P4) and a normal control. The normal spectra are essentially unremarkable. The parkinsonian plots, however, show a principle frequency component at 9.2Hz, with additional peaks at 4.5Hz in the upper lip and at 13.5Hz in all three structures. Spectrally, these postural tremors share the 8.0 to 9.0Hz component with the resting tremor (Figure 3-2). In the upper lip, the major difference is in the relative magnitude of the 4.5 and 9.0Hz component (i.e., the 9.0Hz frequency component is dominant in the postural states while the 4.0 to 5.0Hz frequency component is dominant at rest). The differences in the spectral composition from those in the limbs suggest that orofacial postural tremor might be a partial manifestation of the orofacial resting tremor rather than the result of a totally different tremorogenic mechanism as hypothesized for the spinal system. This partial similarity between the orofacial tremor noted at rest and during posturing might be explained by the fact that the orofacial muscles are not specifically antigravity muscles such as those in the limbs, and, therefore, they may manifest a modified form of resting tremor when voluntarily postured.

Postural tremor is also observed during isometric muscular contractions of different magnitudes. As noted previously, postural tremor recorded under these conditions takes on special diagnostic significance if observations made in the limbs are verified in the orofacial system. That is, if correlation between the rates of (1) firing of motor units, (2) voluntary movements, and (3) tremor during isometric force tasks are found in the orofacial system, it would enhance the significance of isometric force monitoring as a technique to obtain quantitative indices of nervous system integrity. Based on this rationale, similar correlations were sought in the orofacial system, utilizing the custom-designed orofacial force transducers described previously. A sample of the isometric force signals recorded from both parkinsonian and normal control subjects are shown in Figure 3-5. A typical spectral analysis of these static portions of the isometric force signals are shown in Figure 3-6. As is apparent, normal force oscillations showed a dominant spectral peak at 8.5Hz, while parkinsonian force oscillations occurred at 4.0

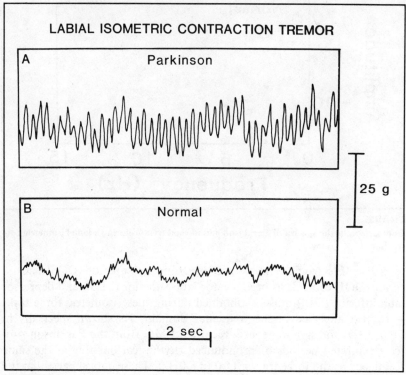

FIGURE 3-5
Tremor oscillographic recordings from a Parkinsonian dysarthric (A) and a normal subject (B) during a labial isometric contraction of 50 grams.

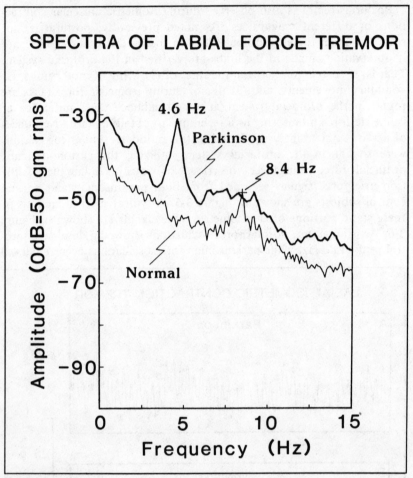

FIGURE 3-6
Comparison of the spectra of Parkinson and normal tremor during a labial isometric contraction of 50 grams.

to 5.0Hz. Electromyographic activity from the superior (OOS) and inferior (OOI) orbicularis oris, levator labii superior (LLS), and depressor labii inferior (DLI) muscles obtained during these isometric force tasks were also analyzed in the frequency domain. As shown spectrally in Figure 3-7, the simultaneously recorded EMG from the Parkinson subjects exhibited periods of pronounced rhythmical bursting at the same frequency as the force tremor (4.0 to 5.0Hz). These data suggest that the correlation in the frequency domain between facial muscle EMG and the generated isometric force tremor is comparable to the relationship pro-

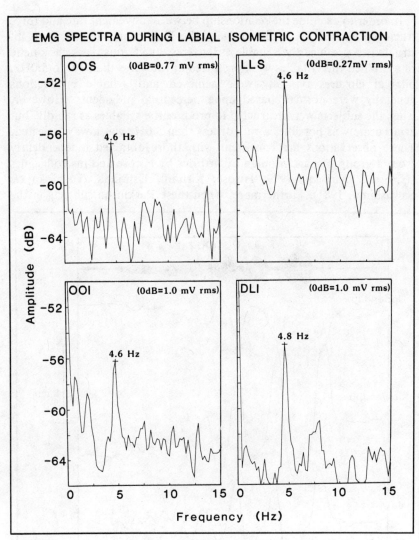

FIGURE 3-7
Spectra of muscle activity from OOS, LLS, OOI, and DLI during a labial isometric contraction of 50 grams from a Parkinson subject.

posed by Freund and Dietz (1978) between the dominant single motor unit firing rate in individual muscles and the dominant frequency in isometric force oscillations. However, this causal relationship has yet to be empirically determined at the single motor unit level in the orofacial system of Parkinson dysarthrics.

In order to examine the relationship between movement rate and force tremor proposed by Freund (1982), the Parkinson subjects were instructed to produce the syllable string /pɑ/ at various diadochokinetic rates. When the syllables were produced at rates less than 4.0 to 5.0Hz, bilabial closures typically were achieved and syllable productions generally were normal, based upon perceptual judgments. However, when the subjects were instructed to produce the syllables as rapidly, but as accurately as possible, a rate of less than 5.0Hz was always selected. These observations are consistent with those obtained independently from a group of parkinsonian dysarthrics by Hirose and his colleagues (Hirose & Kiritani, 1979; Hirose, Kiritani, Ushijima, Yoshioka, & Sawashima, 1981). Furthermore, when these Parkinson subjects in the

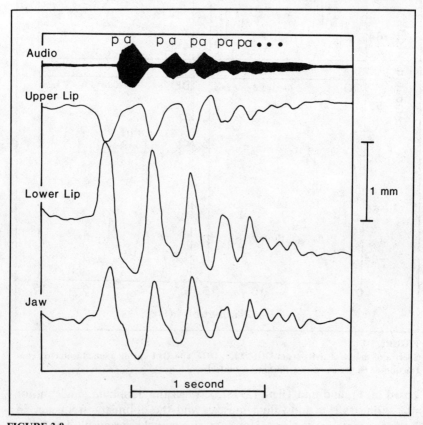

FIGURE 3-8
Oscillographic records of the speech acoustic signal and upper lip, lower lip, and jaw movements during an accelerated production of the syllable string /pɑ/ by a Parkinsonian dysarthric.

present study (with the exception of P1 and P7) were encouraged to exceed the 5.0Hz self-imposed limit, labial movements become markedly reduced in range, and an acceleration or hastening pattern was discernible. An example of such acceleration is shown in Figure 3-8. As is apparent, when this Parkinson subject (P6) exceeded the repetition rate of 5.0Hz, the upper lip, lower lip, and jaw movements effectively become nonfunctional; labial closure was not achieved, due to the reduced range of movement, and glottal abduction for the voiceless stops was absent. These findings suggest that controlled movements cannot exceed the 4.0 to 5.0Hz limit as predicted from the force tremor spectra, and that the phenomenon of acceleration might be related to an aberrant neuromotor system "resonance" at this dominant force tremor frequency. Seemingly, the neural pathways responsible for the isometric force tremors are also implicated in the aberrant movements observed in the parkinsonian population. This potentially significant relationship offers the basis for a number of additional studies in the orofacial system of Parkinson subjects, using tremor spectral analysis in conjunction with parallel observations of speech movement and muscle activity.

STUDY THREE: ACTION TREMOR

Brief rationale. The term action tremor denotes an appendicular tremor which is independent of posture and elicited by voluntary innervation; it is not typically intensified by reinforcement, as is the intention tremor associated with cerebellar disease (Struppler et al., 1978). DeJong (1926) originally described action tremor in the limbs of Parkinson patients and distinguished it from resting tremor because it was triggered by muscle action, either automatic or volitional. Later studies (Andrews et al., 1973; Angel, Aguilar, & Hofmann, 1969; Bishop et al., 1948; Growdon et al., 1975; Lance, Schwab, & Peterson, 1963; Teravainen & Calne, 1980) have confirmed the presence of this tremor during movement, oscillating at a frequency between 7.0 and 12.0Hz. From their observations, Lance et al. (1963) hypothesized a separation of resting and action tremors in parkinsonism as distinct physiological entities because (1) synchronized activation of agonist and antagonist muscles was found during action tremor, while reciprocal activity was evident in resting tremor, and (2) the dominant higher frequency in action tremor was without any apparent harmonic relationship to that of resting tremor. Growdon et al. (1975) confirmed these findings and similarly concluded that action and resting tremor forms are clinically and electromyographically distinct.

More recently, however, the proposed separation between resting and action tremor has become less clear. For example, several investigators have found the patterns of limb EMG activity in Parkinson tremors to be quite variable; i.e., either synchronous or reciprocal activity has been reported in conjunction with both action and resting tremor (Andrews et al., 1973; Bishop et al., 1948; Landau et al., 1966; Teravainen & Calne, 1980). Moreover, with the advent of spectral signal analysis techniques, a harmonic relationship between the low frequency component associated with resting tremor and the high frequency component associated with action tremor has been demonstrated (Dietz et al., 1975; Teravainen & Calne, 1980). In light of these controversial findings in the limbs and the documentation of resting tremor in the orofacial system, it is of interest to examine the orofacial system for manifestations of action tremor and explore its relationship to orofacial resting tremor. Moreover, inasmuch as speech involves the fine control of actions in multiple muscle systems, such tremor, if present, may have a significant negative influence upon speech.

Specific tasks. Action tremor in the orofacial system was observed during the various speech production tasks. The speech sample included the production of the syllable /pɑ/ at (1) a self-defined comfortable rate, (2) controlled rates of 2 per and 4 per sec. and (3) as rapidly, but as accurately as possible. Subjects also produced the sentence, *Buy Bobby a Poppy,* at a normal rate and intensity level.

Observations in the orofacial system. During each of the speech tasks, action tremor was observed in the structures of the orofacial system in each of the Parkinson subjects, with the exception of P8. As is apparent from the sample oscillographic record shown in Figure 3-9, action tremor is superimposed on parkinsonian speech movements. Figure 3-10 shows a representative series of spectral plots from analyses of orofacial movement data from a parkinsonian dysarthric and a normal control during the /pɑ/ production at a rate of approximately 2 per sec. For the dysarthric subjects, a large amplitude 9.2Hz frequency component is present in the spectral plots as well as the lower frequency components associated with the voluntary movement patterns. By comparison, frequency analyses of lip and jaw movement patterns in the normal subjects show spectral peaks only at the voluntary movement frequency. If one compares the spectral observations of action tremor with the spectral plots obtained from analyzing the same structures during the resting condition (Figure 3-2), there is some indication that one of the same frequency components is present in both cases. That is, at rest the 8.0 to 9.0Hz component also is present, but at a lower relative amplitude. It appears that the 8.0 to 9.0Hz frequency component is maintained during both tasks which might support a common pathogenesis for both resting and

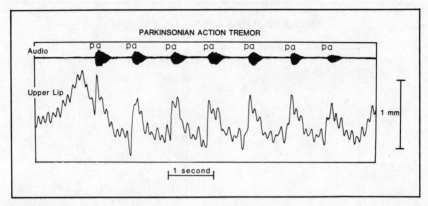

FIGURE 3-9
Oscillographic records of the speech acoustic signal and upper lip movement with superimposed action tremor during the production of the syllable string /pɑ/ by a Parkinsonian dysarthric.

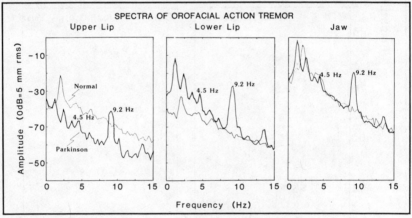

FIGURE 3-10
Comparison of the spectra from a normal (light line) and a Parkinson subject (dark line) for the upper lip, lower lip, and jaw during the production of a sequence of /pɑ/s.

action tremors. Moreover, inspection of EMG records in the time domain did not reveal the proposed differences in EMG patterns for action and resting tremor (i.e., synchronous vs. reciprocal antagonistic muscle activity). However, analysis of these same EMG records in the frequency domain (Figure 3-11) does indicate muscular activity at the movement frequency and at each of the tremor frequencies, tending to support the separate tremorogenic mechanism hypothesis. Further studies comparing normals and Parkinson subjects with various speech and nonspeech

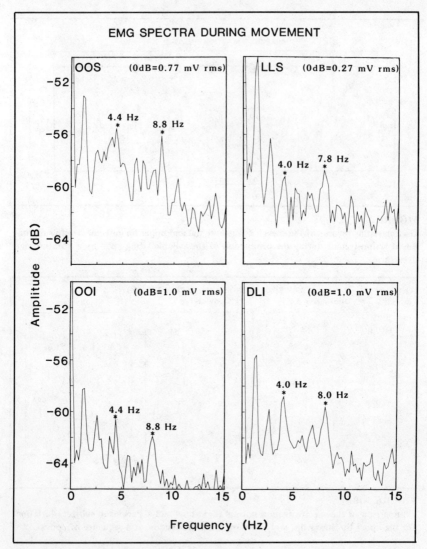

FIGURE 3-11
Spectra of muscle activity from OOS, LLS, OOI, and DLI during the production of a sequence of /pɑ/s by a Parkinsonian dysarthric.

paradigms (i.e., attempting to reset the tremor during rest and speech and/or perturbating a resting structure with various beat frequencies will be required to further test these various "tremor origin" hypotheses) (cf. Lee & Stein, 1981; Walsh, 1979).

STUDY FOUR: COGWHEELING

Brief rationale. It is well known that in passively moving a joint of an affected limb of a parkinsonian patient, one encounters increased resistance (i.e., muscle rigidity). Frequently, this resistance is not smooth throughout the excursion, but increments of resistance are discernible (i.e., the cogwheel effect). Lance et al. (1963) found that the cogwheel phenomena in the limbs represented an oscillatory phenomenon, with frequencies ranging up from those of resting tremor (4.0 to 5.0Hz) to the range for action tremor (8.0 to 9.0Hz). Findley et al. (1981) found one group of Parkinson subjects with a mean cogwheeling frequency of 6.2Hz, indicating that the frequency distribution was biased towards 6.0Hz, similar to that of a hand postural tremor and myoclonic activity about the wrist. A second group of patients exhibited a cogwheeling which ranged in frequency between 7.5 to 9.0Hz with a mean of 8.6Hz, similar to the frequency range of action tremor. This latter type of resistance to passive movement was said to feel smoother and more regular than the lower frequency and was described as "rippling." Based upon the similarity in frequencies, Findley et al. (1981) concluded that distinct forms of cogwheeling may exist that are manifestations of postural tremor, action tremor, or clonus superimposed on rigid muscles.

Specific tasks. In a previous study, muscle rigidity was quantified in the labial muscles of four parkinsonian subjects (P1, P4, P5, P7) by applying known forces and observing the resultant *passive* displacements to determine labial muscle stiffness coefficients (Hunker et al., 1982). This experimental technique not only allowed for quantification of labial rigidity but also provided for the examination of cogwheeling in the labial muscles where abnormal levels of stiffness were observed.

Observations in the orofacial system. The passive labial displacement signals from the parkinsonian dysarthrics and normal controls were subjected to spectral analyses. While the parkinsonian displacements yielded results consistent with the observations of cogwheeling reported by Findley et al. (1981), the normal displacement analyses, by contrast, were unremarkable. Illustrated in Figure 3-12A is a representative spectral plot from one of the Parkinson subjects (P5). The cogwheeling exhibited by this subject was a periodic waveform with a primary spectral peak in the 6.0 to 7.0Hz range. These results are particularly interesting in light of the fact that a dominant tremor frequency within this range was not present during any of the previous experimental conditions. One explanation for this disparate finding is that the passive displacement may have actually evoked a 6.5Hz oscillatory pattern clinically similar to

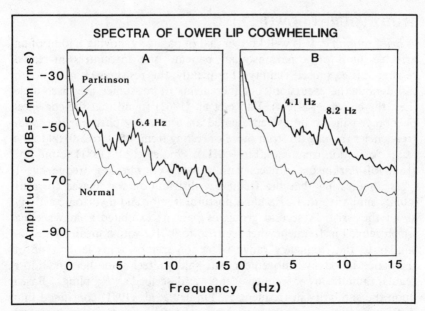

FIGURE 3-12

Comparison of spectra from a normal (light line) and Parkinson subject (dark line) for the lower lip during the passive displacement condition. (A) shows cogwheeling with a primary peak at 6.4Hz and (B) with peaks at 4.1Hz and 8.2Hz.

clonus (i.e., a transient sinusoidal oscillation, which, when imposed on a rigid muscle, is perceived as cogwheeling). This hypothesis was originally proposed by Findley et al. (1981) after comparing wrist supination-pronation clonus with the 6.0Hz cogwheeling and finding similarities in both frequency and time domain analyses. The possible manifestation of myoclonus in the orofacial system as an interpretation of the 6.0 to 7.0Hz cogwheeling phenomena must be investigated further, particularly as it may be manifest during voluntary movements where one muscle group stretches or changes the position of other coupled muscles (e.g., the facial or lingual muscles). For the remaining Parkinson subjects, two distinct spectral peaks were present (4.0 to 4.5Hz and 8.0 to 9.0Hz) (Figure 3-12B). As is apparent, these frequencies are harmonically related, suggestive of the previously observed spectra for resting, postural, and action tremors in the orofacial structures.

DYNAMIC FLUCTUATION OF TREMOR FORMS

As is apparent, distinct pathological tremors were observed in the orofacial system when the structures were at rest, postured, and actively or passively moved. Each of these various tremor forms had dominant frequencies with associated spectral components that fluctuated in their relative amplitudes with variations in the motor performance condition.

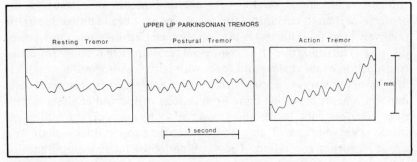

FIGURE 3-13
Oscillograph records of resting tremor, postural tremor, and action tremor in the upper lip of a Parkinsonian dysarthric obtained sequentially within a 20-sec interval.

Figure 3-13 is an oscillographic record of three of these tremor forms present in the upper lip of the same subject (P4) during rest, posturing, and action, each displaying its characteristic oscillatory pattern. Of note is that this particular sequence of resting, postural, and action tremor was manifest within a 20 sec. interval; these distinct tremors were obvious in the upper lip as soon as transitions were made from one motor performance condition to another. Comparable patterns were seen in the lower lip and jaw during a sequence of similar motor performance transitions. These results suggest that the involuntary tremor oscillations of a muscle system (such as the lips) are modified dynamically as a function of motor performance conditions. Dynamic modifications in dominant tremor characteristics (i.e., modulation of relative amplitudes of multiple frequency components) may be due to (1) alterations in biomechanical characteristics (e.g., changes in muscle stiffness with transitions from passive to active states), (2) triggering of alternative tremorogenic pathways or mechanisms, or (3) a combination of these two processes. These factors, as they contribute to modifications in tremor form, may be of particular significance to a more complete understanding of parkinsonian dysarthria. This dynamic, changing quality of Parkinson tremors may be critical during speech production inasmuch as the motor states of the orofacial subsystems are constantly in flux. Hence, different forms of tremor may be present simultaneously in different orofacial structures, each influencing the quality of motor performance in a different manner.

GENERAL DISCUSSION

Based on the observations presented in this paper, it is apparent that earlier considerations on the presence and nature of tremor in the orofacial system of parkinsonian dysarthrics have been limited due to the relatively insensitive measures used to characterize this speech movement disorder. The utilization of instrumental techniques that allow for direct transduction of movement and force with parallel observation of muscle activity apparently is necessary to observe and quantify this potentially important neuromuscular sign. Applications of spectral analysis techniques to movements, forces and associated EMG supports the aforementioned suggestion that it may be inappropriate to consider tremor as a single frequency oscillation. The examination of relative amplitudes of the multiple frequency tremor components may be essential to characterize differences or progressive changes within or among Parkinson patients or to discern possible causal relations between tremor patterns and aberrations of movement.

Particularly interesting is that with direct observation, one finds not only the characteristic resting tremor in these Parkinson subjects, but also other forms of tremor associated with posture and movements of the speech production system. Spectrally, the complex involuntary oscillations present during the various motoric conditions are overlapping in frequency composition, fluctuating primarily in relative amplitude. Hence, the so-called resting tremor may not, as traditionally suggested, disappear during posturing or on initiation of action, but rather may be only reduced in relative amplitude. Similarly, the action temor may not be reflexively triggered by voluntary innervation, but rather is present at rest and is enhanced by voluntary contraction, yielding a more dominant 8.0 to 9.0Hz component. These observations tend to suggest that the involuntary oscillations associated with parkinsonism are spectrally complex, and that particular motoric behavior, with associated biomechanical and neurophysiological differences, transform the tremor waveform so that selected frequency components become dominant. Although this is obviously an oversimplification of the issues concerning the pathogenesis of the various tremor forms, it is a fruitful basis for further investigation. Such investigations, if carefully conducted, may yield some sensitive indices for differential subgrouping of Parkinson dysarthrics and provide further indications of the central nervous system pathways that may be involved in any given subject.

Neuroanatomical Sources of Tremor

Despite large numbers of clinical and scientific studies, the origin of the various pathological tremors in Parkinson's disease remains unclear.

One explanation for these tremors, increasingly proposed in recent years, is based on the notion of central oscillators. Hypothetically, these mechanisms can take many forms, such as a single cell which has an intrinsic rhythm, as in the case of cardiac cells (pacemakers), or an interconnection between cells that yield oscillations (network oscillations). A simple example of this latter model is the negative feedback network of Renshaw cells on to motoneurons or of thalamic cells on to cortical cells. The general consistency of tremor patterns for the cranial and spinal systems, as noted in this chapter, supports a central oscillatory network as the principal basis for the tremors symptomatic of Parkinson's disease. The apparent result of the dopaminergic imbalance in the basal ganglia of parkinsonian patients is the synchronized firing of motoneurons to a rhythm of 4.0 to 5.0Hz. This has been demonstrated in the limbs (cf. Freund & Dietz, 1978) and in the orofacial system in the present series of studies. Since parkinsonian tremor only occurs in the waking state, the most likely source of synchronization is through the cortex via the corticobulbar/spinal pathways. Furthermore, elimination of tremor can be obtained by removing the afferent input to the motor cortex at thalamic nuclei where dentatothalamic fibers terminate (Hassler, Mundinger, & Riechert, 1970). This observation has provided the basis for thalamic lesions as a therapeutic procedure for tremor relief. Based upon this logic, a central oscillatory network theory involving known cerebellar-thalamic-cortical-spinal pathways has evolved as a potential tremorogenic mechanism for spinal systems tremor. That is, the basic argument is that altercation of basal ganglion input to the thalamus in Parkinson's disease leads to an oscillatory pattern within this proposed suprasegmental network (Calne, 1970; Evarts, Teravainen, Beuchert, & Calne, 1979; Hassler et al., 1970). Since analyses of tremor in the orofacial system have provided results comparable to those obtained from the limbs, one might predict that the same network is responsible for cranial system tremor.

Possible Significance of Tremor in Speech Movement Disorders

The presence of tremors during almost all of the states of the speech production movement process may have significant implications for some of the speech motor deficits associated with this disease. For example, during many speech utterances, some parts of the system are effectively in states of posturing (respiratory system, larynx, velum, and so on) while others are transiently at rest, while yet other muscle systems (especially the articulators) are involved in various "actions." If the tremors associated with these various conditions influence movement control, their disparate influence may be fluctuating from one moment of the system's actions to another, depending on the speech task-dependent conditions of the subsystems. For example, for some speech sequences the jaw might maintain a posture with minimal movement actions while during other sequences discrete "actions" of the jaw may be required; comparable variations in movement behavior as a function of speech task requirements are certain to be present for almost all speech motor subsystems. If these various tremor forms have different aberrant influences on movement control, it is possible that the specific movement disorders associated with parkinsonian dysarthria dynamically change across speech subsystems as a function of their moment-to-moment motor performance requirements.

The potential significance of tremor as a causal factor in the movement aberrations seen in the parkinsonian population has yielded several specific hypotheses, at least one of which was supported directly with data presented in the present study. Data from several studies (Draper & Johns, 1964; Evarts, Teravainen, & Calne, 1981; Hallett & Khoshbin, 1980) suggest that alterations in the duration and velocity of limb movements (e.g., bradykinesia) seen in Parkinson subjects may be attributed, at least to some degree, to the interference of tremor. For example, it has been suggested that the prolonged reaction times seen in Parkinson subjects may be due to an inability to initiate a contraction until it coincides with the involuntary quasi-rhythmic, excitatory-agonistic burst of a tremor oscillation. If, as noted, the resting tremor has a prominent spectral component at 4.0 to 6.0Hz and the stimulus for initiation of a reaction time is random with respect to the inhibitory/excitatory tremor cycle, one might predict an average increase in reaction time ranging from 90 to 125 msec. These calculations have been substantiated empirically in Parkinson subjects in the observation of prolonged reaction times by Evarts et al. (1981) and others. If the same limitation is imposed upon time-critical movements for speech, delays of this magnitude would be quite detrimental to actions such as initiation of vocal fold adduction (re: the generation of appropriate voice onset times), temporal intermovement timing for certain consonant clusters, and so on. It would be useful to examine movement and muscle patterns during speech of Parkinson dysarthrics to discern the nature and degree of intermuscle and movement variability in relation to possible tremor-induced aberrations. In this vein, it is interesting that for many Parkinson dysarthrics where accelerometer measures of vocal fold vibration have been obtained, there often is an absence of normal voiceless intervals. If certain movements such as rapid adduction/abduction of vocal folds cannot be made within a 90 to 125 msec time, they may be eliminated as a compensatory necessity.

Observations of Hallett and Khoshbin (1980) offer yet another suggestion for a causal relation between movement aberrations and tremor. Their data suggest that movement time is prolonged due to the superimposition of a number of tremor-related agonist/antagonist inhibitions. These periodic excitatory inhibitory volleys bear a strong resemblance to action tremor, silencing the muscle periodically and, hence, reducing the overall movement velocity. Rather than having a single velocity peak, movements are multisloped, corresponding to the excitatory-inhibitory periods. Likewise, Draper and Johns (1964) observed plateaus during limb movement trajectories with corresponding multiple velocity peaks. The explanation offered from these observations was that the periodic, inhibitory interference of action tremor actually prolonged the duration of the movement. The patterns of movement shown in Figure 3-9 would support this interpretation.

Finally are the observations in the present study and the suggestions of Freund (1982) that the force tremor spectral peak seen during isometric contractions is a reflection of the inability to recruit large motoneurons below their tonic threshold, hence limiting movement velocities and the associated maximum rate of voluntary movement. Apparently this is reflected in the approximately 4.0Hz limit at which many parkinsonian subjects can produce rapid alternating speech movements. Potentially, the manifestation of this apparent limitation on motoneuron recruitment rates could reflect the slowness of parkinsonian speech. Moreover, given disparate motoneuron composition for the jaw, tongue, lips, and so on, such a limitation may be non-uniform in its influences for different speech motor subsystems.

Clinical Significance

Overall, these hypotheses concerning the potential motor impairment significance of tremor in Parkinson subjects suggest a number of fruitful applied clinical efforts. For example, based upon the observations of Evarts et al. (1981) and Hallett and Khoshbin (1980), one should be able to predict the degree and nature of bradykinesia from observations of tremor spectra and the relative amplitude of tremor components. Further, observations on prominent spectral components of isometric force generation such as those of Freund (1982) should allow one to predict movement limitations for speech or individual structural movements. For example, if spectral peaks in isometric forces of the tongue were different than those in the lips (cf. Abbs et al., 1983), maximum diadochokinetic rates for [pɑ] should be different than those for [tɑ].

In this regard, the potential clinical utility of tremor analyses appears substantial. In terms of assessment, quantification of tremor spectra from the various speech motor subsystems may offer an objective means of determining the relative degree of impairment in those subsystems individually, and thus a basis from which to predict associated speech movement aberrations. That is, these analyses, given the relative ease with which they can be conducted, may permit pathophysiological interpretation of speech output aberrations that have been observed more globally with other measures. For example, observations of isometric force tremors in the tongue would allow one to specifically explain lingual articulation breakdowns at speech rates exceeding the primary tremor frequency. By contrast, the absence of parallel aberrant tremors in the labial musculature would explain the paradoxical observations of relatively normal productions of labial articulations in the same subject. In this regard, it would be interesting also to examine the hypothesized progression of motor impairment across speech motor subsystems (cf. Logemann, Fisher, Boshes, & Blonsky, 1978) utilizing these more refined analysis techniques. These measures also would provide sensitive indices as to the influence of certain therapy programs, including pharmacological as well as behavioral regimens. One might even consider using behavioral techniques like biofeedback in conjunction with a real-time spectrum analyzer to determine whether Parkinson's disease patients can reduce the amplitude of tremor components that interfere with voluntary movement.

Finally, there would appear to be significant value in utilizing tremor analyses under different motor performance conditions and among orofacial and limb subsystems as a basis for more refined subclassification of individuals with Parkinson's disease. The presence and degree of tremors among motor subsystems for resting, postural/isometric, and action states may offer an objective means for specifying Parkinson's disease subgroups and determining in parallel which central neural pathways are impaired (cf. Evarts et al., 1979; Hassler et al., 1970). That is, due to the somatotopic organization of the basal ganglia, one would not predict uniform tremor manifestations across orofacial and limb motor subsystems; to the extent that these manifestations are nonuniform, involvement of certain nuclei and pathways could be hypothesized, at least in a functional sense (cf. Grimm & Nashner, 1978). With improved subclassification of parkinsonian dysarthrics, prognosis and specification of optimal treatment should be improved.

REFERENCES

Abbs, J. H., Hunker, C. J., & Barlow, S. M. Differential speech motor subsystem impairments in subjects with suprabulbar lesions: Neurophysiological framework and supporting data. In W. Berry (Ed.), *Clinical dysarthria*. San Diego: College-Hill Press, 1983, 21-56.

Abbs, J. H., & Muller, E. M. *Neurophysiological and biomechanical factors in articulatory movement*. Paper presented at the Conference on the Production of Speech, Austin, TX, 1980.

Abbs, J. H., Sutton, D., Larson, C., & Eilenberg, G. R. *Neuromuscular mechanisms underlying speech production (Program Project NINCDS NS11780)*. Seattle: University of Washington, 1973.

Allum, J. H. J., Dietz, V., & Freund, H.-J. Neuronal mechanisms underlying physiological tremor. *Journal of Neurophysiology*, 1978, *41*, 557-571.

Andrews, C. J., Burke, D., & Lance, J. W. The comparison of tremors in normal, parkinsonian, and athetotic man. *Journal of the Neurological Sciences*, 1973, *19*, 53-61.

Angel, R. W., Aguilar, J. A., & Hofmann, W. W. Action tremor and thalamotomy. *Electroencephalography and Clinical Neurophysiology*, 1969, *26*, 80-85.

Barlow, S. M., & Abbs, J. H. Force transducers for the evaluation of labial, lingual, and mandibular function in dysarthria. *Journal of Speech and Hearing Research*, in press.

Barlow, S. M., Cole, K. J., & Abbs, J. H. A new headmounted lip-jaw movement transduction system for the study of motor speech disorders. *Journal of Speech and Hearing Research*, 1983, *26*, 283-288.

Bishop, G. H., Clare, M. H., & Price, J. Patterns of tremor in normal and pathological conditions. *Journal of Applied Physiology*, 1948, *1*, 123-147.

Calne, D. B. *Parkinsonism: Physiology, pharmacology and treatment*. London: Edward Arnold, 1970.

Calne, D. B., & Lader, M. H. Electromyographic studies of tremor using an averaging computer. *Electroencephalography and Clinical Neurophysiology*, 1969, *26*, 86-92.

Darley, F. L., Aronson, A. E., & Brown, J. R. Differential diagnostic patterns of dysarthria. *Journal of Speech and Hearing Research*, 1969, *12*, 246-269. (a)

Darley, F. L., Aronson, A. E., & Brown, J. R. Clusters of deviant speech dimensions in the dysarthrias. *Journal of Speech and Hearing Research*, 1969, *12*, 462-496. (b)

Darley, F. L., Aronson, A. E., & Brown, J. R. *Motor speech disorders*. Philadelphia: Saunders, 1975.

Dejerine, J. *Séméilogie des affections du système nerveus*. Paris: Masson, 1914.

DeJong, H. Action-tremor. *Journal of Nervous and Mental Diseases*, 1926, *64*, 1-11.

Desmedt, J. E. (Ed.). *Progress in clinical neurophysiology* (10 vols.). Basel: Karger, 1973-1982.

Desmedt, J. E. (Ed.). *Physiological tremor, pathological tremors and clonus*. Basel: Karger, 1978.

Dietrichson, P., Engebretsen, O., Fonstelien, E., & Hovland, J. Quantifiction of tremor in man. In J. E. Desmedt (Ed.), *Physiological tremor, pathological tremors and clonus*. Basel: Karger, 1978, 90-94.

Dietz, V., Bischofberger, E., Wita, C., & Freund, H.-J. Correlation between the discharges of two simultaneously recorded motor units and physiological tremor. *Electroencephalography and Clinical Neurophysiology,* 1976, *40,* 97-105.

Dietz, V., Freund, H.-J., & Allum, J. H. J. Parkinsonian tremor during rest and voluntary contraction and its correlation with single motor unit activity. In W. Birkmayer & O. Hornykiewicz (Eds.), *Advances in parkinsonism: Biochemistry, physiology, treatment.* Basel: Roche, 1975, 244-250.

Dietz, V., Hillesheimer, W., & Freund, H.-J. Correlation between tremor, voluntary contraction, and firing pattern of motor units in Parkinson's disease. *Journal of Neurology, Neurosurgery, and Psychiatry,* 1974, *37,* 927-937.

Draper, I. T., & Johns, R. J. The disordered movement in parkinsonism and the effect of drug treatment. *Bulletin of Johns Hopkins Hospital,* 1964, *115,* 465-480.

Elble, R. J., & Randall, J. E. Motor-unit activity responsible for 8- to 12-Hz component of human physiological finger tremor. *Journal of Neurophysiology,* 1976, *39,* 370-383.

Evarts, E. V., Teravainen, H. T., Beuchert, D. E., & Calne, D. B. Pathophysiology of motor performance in Parkinson's disease. In D. Calne & K. Fuxe (Eds.), *Dopaminergic ergot derivatives and motor functions.* Oxford: Pergamon, 1979, 45-59.

Evarts, E. V., Teravainen, H., & Calne, D. B. Reaction time in Parkinson's disease. *Brain,* 1981, *104,* 167-186.

Findley, L. J., Gresty, M. A., & Halmagyi, G. M. Tremor, the cogwheel phenomenon and clonus in Parkinson's disease. *Journal of Neurology, Neurosurgery, and Psychiatry,* 1981, *44,* 534-546.

Freund, H.-J. Pathophysiological basis of some voluntary motor disorders. In B. Petterson & W. Zev Rymer (Chairs), *International Conference on the Neurophysiological Basis of Motor Disorders.* Chicago: Rehabilitation Institute of Chicago, 1982.

Freund, H.-J., Budingen, H. J., & Dietz, V. Activity of single motor units from human forearm muscles during voluntary isometric contractions. *Journal of Neurophysiology,* 1975, *38,* 933-946.

Freund, H.-J., & Dietz, V. The relationship between physiological and pathological tremor. In J. E. Desmedt (Ed.), *Physiological tremor, pathological tremor and clonus.* Basel: Karger, 1978, 66-89.

Freund, H.-J., Dietz, V., Wita, C.W., & Kapp, H. Discharge characteristics of single motor units in normal subjects and patients with supraspinal motor disturbances. In J. E. Desmedt (Ed.), *New developments in electromyography and clinical neurophysiology.* Basel: Karger, 1973, 242-250.

Grimm, R. J., & Nashner, L. M. Long loop dyscontrol. In J. E. Desmedt (Ed.), *Cerebral motor control in man: Long loop mechanisms.* Basel: Karger, 1978, 70-84.

Growden, J. H., Young, R. R., & Shahani, B. T. The differential diagnosis of tremor in Parkinson's disease. *Transactions of the American Neurological Association,* 1975, *100,* 197-199.

Hallett, M., & Khoshbin, S. The physiological mechanism of bradykinesia. *Brain,* 1980, *163,* 301-314.

Hassler, R., Mundinger, F., & Riechert, T. Pathophysiology of tremor at rest derived from the correlation of anatomical and clinical data. *Confinia Neurologica,* 1970, *32,* 79-87.

Hirose, H., & Kiritani, S. Velocity of articulatory movements in normal and dysarthric subjects. *Annual Bulletin of the Research Institute of Logopedics and Phoniatrics,* 1979, *13,* 105-112.

Hirose, H., Kiritani, S., Ushijima, T., Yoshioka, H., & Sawashima, M. Patterns of dysarthric movements in patients with parkinsonism. *Folia Phoniatrica,* 1981, *33,* 204-215.

Hunker, C. J., Abbs, J. H. & Barlow, S. M. The relationship between parkinsonian rigidity and hypokinesia in the orofacial system: A quantitative analysis. *Neurology,* 1982, *32,* 749-754.

Kennedy, J. G., & Abbs, J. H. Anatomical studies of the perioral motor system: Foundations for studies in speech pathology. In N. J. Lass (Ed.), *Speech and language: Advances in basic research and practice* (Vol. 1). New York: Academic Press, 1979, 211-270.

Konopacki, R. A., & Cole, K. J. Evaluation of electrodes for speech muscle electromyography. *Journal of the Acoustical Society of America* (Suppl. 1), 1982, *71,* S33.

Lance, J. W., Schwab, R. S., & Peterson, E. A. Action tremor and the cogwheel phenomena in Parkinson's disease. *Brain,* 1963, *86,* 95-110.

Landau, W. M., Struppler, A., & Mehls, O. A comparative electromyographic study of the reactions to passive movement in parkinsonism and in normal subjects. *Neurology,* 1966, *16,* 34-48.

Lee, R. G., & Stein, R. B. Resetting of tremor by mechanical perturbations: A comparison of essential tremor and parkinsonian tremor. *Annals of Neurology,* 1981, *10,* 525-531.

Logemann, J. A., Fisher, H. B., Boshes, B., & Blonsky, E. Frequency and co-occurrence of vocal tract dysfunctions in the speech of a large sample of Parkinson patients. *Journal of Speech and Hearing Disorders,* 1978, *43,* 47-57.

Marsden, C. D. The mechanisms of physiological tremor and their significance for pathological tremors. In J. E. Desmedt (Ed.), *Physiological tremor, pathological tremors and clonus.* Basel: Karger, 1978, 1-16.

Milner-Brown, H. S., Fisher, M. A., & Weiner, W. J. Electrical properties of motor units in parkinsonism and a possible relationship with bradykinesia. *Journal of Neurology, Neurosurgery, and Psychiatry,* 1979, *42,* 35-41.

Milner-Brown, H. S., Stein, R. B., & Yemm, R. The contractile properties of human motor units during voluntary isometric contractions. *Journal of Physiology,* 1973, *228,* 285-306.

Müller, E. M., & Macleod, G. Perioral biomechanics and its relation to labial motor control. *Journal of Acoustical Society of America* (Suppl. 1), 1982, *71,* S33.

Rack, P. M. H. Mechanical and reflex factors in human tremor. In J. E. Desmedt (Ed.), *Physiological tremor, pathological tremors and clonus.* Basel: Karger, 1978, 17-27.

Rondot, P., Jedynak, C. P., & Ferrey, G. Pathological tremors: Nosological correlates. In J. E. Desmedt (Ed.), *Physiological tremor, pathological tremors and clonus.* Basel: Karger, 1978, 95-113.

Stalberg, E., & Young, R. R. *Clinical neurophysiology.* Boston: Butterworths International Medical Reviews, 1981.

Stein, R. B., & Lee, R. G. Tremor and clonus. In V. B. Brooks (Ed.), *Handbook of physiology, Section 1* (Vol. 2: Motor control, Part 1). Bethesda, MD: American Physiological Society, 1981, 325-344.

Stiles, R. N., & Pozos, R. S. A mechanical-reflex oscillator hypothesis for parkinsonian hand tremor. *Journal of Applied Physiology,* 1976, *40,* 990-998.

Struppler, A., Erbel, F., & Velho, F. An overview on the pathophysiology of parkinsonian and other pathological tremor. In J. E. Desmedt (Ed.), *Physiological tremor, pathological tremors and clonus.* Basel: Karger, 1978, 114-128.

Teravainen, H., & Calne, D. B. Action tremor in Parkinson's disease. *Journal of Neurology, Neurosurgery, and Psychiatry,* 1980, *43,* 257-263.

Wachs, H., & Boshes, B. Tremor studies in normals and in parkinsonism. *Archives of Neurology,* 1961, *4,* 66-82.

Walsh, E. G. Beats produced between a rhythmic applied force and the resting tremor of parkinsonism. *Journal of Neurology, Neurosurgery, and Psychiatry,* 1979, *42,* 89-94.

ACKNOWLEDGMENTS

The authors wish to express their gratitude to Dr. Henry Peters of the Departments of Neurology and Rehabilitative Medicine of the University of Wisconsin Clinical Health Sciences Center and the Medical School for granting accessibility to the patients under his care in the Parkinson Clinic. Appreciation is also expressed to Marilyn Parnell for her editorial assistance during the preparation of this manuscript. This work was supported by NINCDS Grant NS13274 and NICHD Grant HD-03352.

4

Articulatory Characteristics of Parkinsonian Dysarthria: Segmental and Phrase-Level Timing, Spirantization, and Glottal-Supraglottal Coordination

Gary Weismer

INTRODUCTION

The articulatory disorder associated with Parkinson's disease is often said to be characterized mainly by imprecise consonant production (Darley, Aronson, & Brown, 1969a, 1969b, 1975). Efforts to specify in greater detail the nature of this imprecision have taken the form of fine-grained perceptual analyses as well as physiological and acoustic descriptions. Logemann and Fisher (1981) concluded from a detailed phonetic analysis that manner errors were most characteristic of parkinsonian dysarthria, the most typical example of which was spirantization of stops. Other perceptual and acoustical analyses (Canter, 1965; Kent & Netsell, 1979; Kent & Rosenbek, 1982) appear to be consistent with this view.

Physiological analyses (Hirose, Kiritani, & Sawashima, 1982; Hirose, Kiritani, Ushijima, Yoshioka, & Sawashima, 1981; Hunker, Abbs, & Barlow, 1982; Leanderson, Persson, & Öhman, 1970) suggest that persons with Parkinson's disease have reduced articulatory displacements relative to normal speakers and improper coordination of agonist-antagonist muscle pairs or groups. This would lead one to suspect that vowel production might also be affected in Parkinson's disease, but relevant data seem to consist only of observations from a single case study (Lehiste, 1965).

The purpose of this chapter is to report a relatively fine-grained temporal analysis of parkinsonian dysarthria. A major motivation for pursuing this type of analysis is the suggestion by some authors that certain aspects of motor programming are disturbed in Parkinson's disease (see summary in DeLong & Georgopoulos, 1981). Timing is often thought to be an integral part of motor programs (Semjen, 1977), and at least one alleged disorder of speech motor programming — apraxia of speech — has been shown to be characterized by aberrant timing (Kent & Rosenbek, 1983). Various authors have commented at least on the gross speaking rate characteristics of parkinsonian dysarthria (Canter, 1963; Critchley, 1981; Darley et al., 1975), noting either unusually slow or fast rates among certain patients. A more detailed examination of the temporal structure of parkinsonian dysarthria seems warranted, therefore, both to improve our understanding of the relationship between the central nervous system pathology and the speech disorder and to formulate more specific hypotheses for the speech physiologist. The present data were obtained by means of acoustic analysis techniques, which have been successfully applied to other speech disorders as well as to normal speech (Kent & Forner, 1980; Weismer & Elbert, 1982; Weismer & Fromm, 1983).

METHODS

Subjects

Three groups of male subjects were studied; two could be considered "control" groups, with the remaining group defined as the "experimental" group. One control group included five young adults, ranging in age from 21 to 27 years. The second control group included eight geriatric adults where "geriatric" was defined as any person 65 years of age or older (the latter subjects ranged in age from 65 to 82 and were free of any known disease states). The third group consisted of eight persons diagnosed medically as having Parkinson's disease, ranging in age from 51 to 83. Subject information is reported in Table 4-1. Note that no special effort was made to match precisely the ages of geriatric and Parkinson's subjects, or to control Parkinson etiology or length and severity of illness. All Parkinson subjects were being treated with some form of dopaminergic medication. In addition, the only auditory

TABLE 4-1
Subject characteristics, including age for all older subjects and length of illness and suspected etiology for Parkinson subjects.
PEP = Postencephalitic, IP = Idiopathic.

	Parkinson Patients			Geriatrics	
Subject	Age	Years Since Diagnosis	Suspected Etiology	Subject	Age
A	51	3	PEP	A	65
B	52	7	PEP	B	67
C	58	1	IP	C	68
D	58	4	PEP	D	72
E	62	10	PEP	E	72
F	63	14	PEP	F	72
G	75	6	IP	G	80
H	83	7	IP	H	82

criterion for inclusion in the study was that subjects be able to produce accurate repetitions of recorded sentences when the peaks of speech energy ranged between 70 to 80dB SPL, at a distance of 1.2 meters from the source.

The geriatric control group was included for two reasons. First, as Parkinson's disease is more prevalent among geriatric adults than among middle-aged and young adults, it is important to be able to determine characteristics of parkinsonian articulation which are typical of the pathology as opposed to the normal aging process. Second, Parkinson's disease may be characterized by certain neurohistological and behavioral changes which may look like exaggerated aging effects (e.g., Appel, 1981; see also McGeer & McGeer, 1975; Petajan & Jarcho, 1975). The utility of this hypothesis for speech production research may be assessed by determining if empirically demonstrated differences in the articulation of normal geriatric and young adults (see Weismer & Fromm, 1983) are exaggerated when Parkinson patients are included in the comparison. This issue is considered in greater detail in the Discussion.

Procedure and Apparatus

The procedure for each subject was to repeat a preconstructed set of sentences under two conditions. For the first condition, subjects were asked to produce the sentences "in a conversational style", whereas, the second condition required subjects to produce the sentences at a speaking rate they considered to be twice as fast as their conversational rate. The "fast rate" condition was always administered after the conversational condition; data from the former condition will not be presented here.

The sentence sets were recorded by having subjects sit in an audiometric booth and wear a head-mounted, directional microphone (Shure SM10A) connected to a tape deck (Teac A-6100) located outside the booth. Mouth-to-microphone distance was held constant within and across subjects at 9 cm. A second tape deck (Pioneer CT-F8282) outside the booth delivered the recorded sentences to subjects via a loudspeaker mounted inside the booth. Subjects were instructed to listen to an entire sentence and then simply repeat the utterance. Gross repetition errors, including lexical errors, yawns, sneezes, and coughs during an utterance, were responded to by resetting the stimulus tape to the sentence in question and obtaining another repetition. Such errors occurred on 1.8% of the sentences produced by geriatric adults, 2.1% of the sentences produced by Parkinson patients, and did not occur among young adults. The intersentence interval on the stimulus tape was approximately 5 sec.

The speech sample was made up of 16 sentences, each occurring five times throughout a randomly ordered set of 80 sentences. The present analysis is based on four of these sentences, including *I took a spoon and dish, The sunlight strikes raindrops in the air, The new socks feel good on my feet,* and *Buy Bobby a puppy.*

Data Analysis

Data analysis consisted of speech waveform duration measurements derived from storage oscilloscope (Tektronix 5103N) displays. Most measurements were made at a sweep speed of 50 msec/division, but a 20 msec/division sweep speed was used when certain decisions required a more detailed display of waveform characteristics. All measurements were made by the author. Remeasurement of a total of 100 waveforms from subjects in each group yielded an average measurement error for segment durations of 5.8 msec. The measurement error tended to be greater for Parkinson and geriatric subjects than for young adults — a finding consistent with previous demonstrations of larger measurement errors for waveforms produced by subjects with speech disorders (Weismer, Dinnsen, & Elbert, 1981; Weismer & Elbert, 1982).

Two types of measurements were obtained. The first type was a conventional type of *segment duration* measure, where interval durations are determined by operationally defining the interval boundaries.[1] The second type of measurement was of a more qualitative nature, involving decisions of (1) whether or not closure intervals of stop consonants were spirantized and (2) whether or not vocal fold vibration continued for more than 20 msec following the supraglottal constriction for a voiceless stop.

Because these qualitative decisions must sometimes be based on subtle waveform characteristics, a conservative approach was adopted in identifying segments as "spirantized" or "voiced for more than 20 msec into a voiceless constriction." Figure 4-1 presents a set of waveforms and the associated spirantization decisions, and Figure 4-2 presents a set of waveforms for the "continued vocal fold vibration" decisions. Spirantization decisions were based on the appearance of the waveform trace corresponding to the stop closure interval. Because the recordings were made under extremely quiet conditions and with low-noise recording equipment, the closure interval of stop consonants produced with a nonleaking supraglottal constriction appeared on the oscilloscope as a flat, thin line. An example of this kind of waveform, classified as "not spirantized," is provided in panel A of Figure 4-1. For a stop to be classified as "spirantized," some thickening of the closure interval trace had to be observed, the presumption being that the thickening corresponds to the aperiodic energy associated with a leaking (fricated) stop constriction. Examples of stops classified as "spirantized" are presented

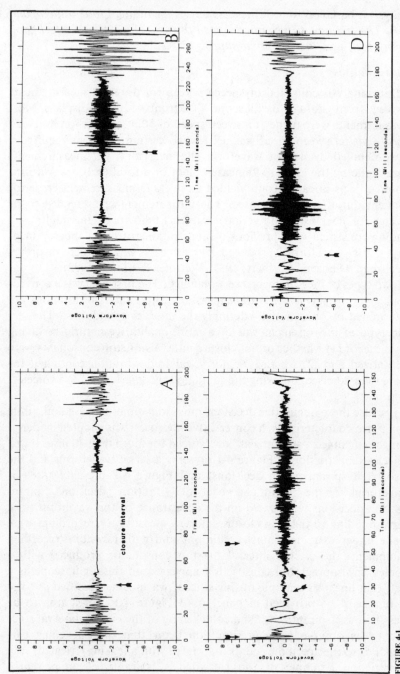

FIGURE 4-1

Selected waveforms illustrating the spirantization decisions made for voiceless stops. Panel A shows a waveform judged to be "nonspirantized," whereas panels B, C, and D show various examples of waveforms judged as "spirantized". In each panel the left hand arrow indicates the onset of the closure interval, and in panels A and B the right hand arrow indicates the stop burst. The raised arrows in panels C and D indicate spirantized portions of the waveforms.

in Figures 4-1B, C, D, where it can be seen that some decisions were based on subtle thickening of the baseline, e.g., panel B, and others on more obvious displays, panels C and D. The waveforms in Figure 4-1 are all associated with voiceless stops, for which the kinds of subtle decisions exemplified in Figure 4-1 B can be made reliably. In the case of voiced stops, the vibrations throughout the closure interval prevent reliable identification of subtle spirantization, but more obvious cases can be identified.

Decisions regarding continuation of vocal fold vibration for more than 20 msec into a voiceless constriction were based on certain waveform characteristics in the vicinity of the vowel-consonant interface. An oscillographic display of voicing during an obstruent typically shows the periodic waveform to be of lesser amplitude than the surrounding vowel; moreover, the waveform associated with each glottal pulse in an obstruent interval will appear to have a less complex shape than corresponding waveforms associated with a vowel. These typical displays are evident in Figure 4-2A, where the amplitude and shape of each cycle in the obstruent interval and vowel intervals are clearly different. These differences can be explained in terms of the way sound is transmitted to an air microphone when the vocal tract is partially or completely obstructed as compared to open. When vocal fold vibration occurs and the vocal tract is partially or completely obstructed, the energy associated with each glottal pulse and its vocal tract response is greatly attenuated relative to the situation when the vocal tract is open; this is why oscillographic displays show such small amplitude glottal pulses during an obstruent interval. Moreover, much or all of the periodic vibration sensed by an air microphone during vocal tract obstruction is transmitted by vibration of the vocal tract *walls,* which act as a low pass filter and thus "reject" much of the higher frequency energy in the glottal spectrum. Thus, the periodic vibrations recorded during the obstruent interval are acoustically less complex than the periodic vibrations associated with vowel production, for which the vocal tract vibrations are transmitted to the microphone mainly via air. This explains the less complex appearance of periodic vibrations during obstruent intervals, as compared to vowels (Figure 4-2A).

These considerations were used in the case of voiceless consonants to decide which vibrations were assigned to the "closed vocal tract interval," and which to the "open vocal tract interval" (that is, the vowel). There are many cases in which voicing apparently ceases at the instant of supraglottal constriction, as illustrated by Figure 4-2B; these would be judged as having no continuation of voicing into the voiceless constriction. Other waveforms show low-amplitude, simple-shaped

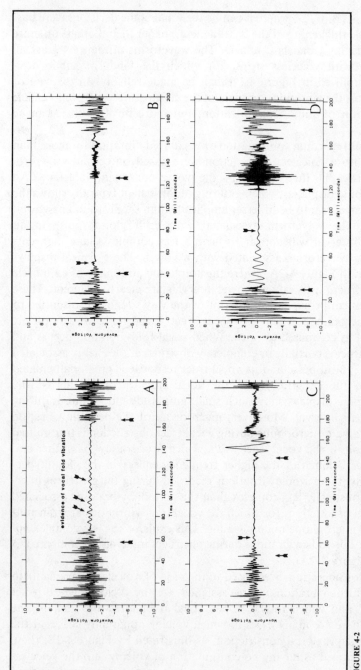

FIGURE 4-2

Selected waveforms illustrating the ''voicing into voiceless closure'' decisions made for voiceless stops. Panel A shows a waveform of a vowel-/b/ = vowel utterance, illustrating difference in amplitude and shape of glottal pulses within the closure interval as compared to during the vowel. Panels B and C show waveforms where voicing does not continue more than 20 msec into the closure interval, whereas panel D shows a waveform where voicing does continue for more than 20 msec. The lower left and right hand arrows in each panel indicate the stop closure and stop burst respectively. In panels B, C and D the downward pointing arrow indicates the offset of vocal fold vibration.

pulses for approximately 20 msec following the final, large amplitude pulse, as shown in Figure 4-2C; these would not meet the present criterion, and so would be grouped with waveforms of the Figure 4-2B type. Finally, waveforms which showed glottal pulses continuing into the voiceless constriction for greater than 20 msec were grouped apart from the type of waveforms shown in Figures 4-2B and 4-2C. For this report, only the binary decisions of whether or not voicing continued for more than 20 msec were recorded. No effort was made to record the time course of the voicing continuation, with the exception of those voiceless consonants which showed voicing throughout the entire constriction interval. This analysis focused on voiceless stops, because the frication energy associated with voiceless fricatives visually masks the glottal pulses that may occur in the constriction interval. An occasional exception to this is /f/, which is produced by most speakers as an extremely weak-intensity fricative.

RESULTS

Segment Durations

Summaries of the results on segment durations are presented graphically in Figures 4-3 through Figure 4-9. In each of these figures, data are plotted for the Parkinson, geriatric adults, and young adult subjects from left to right on the abscissa. Each unfilled data point represents the mean duration of a particular segment for an individual subject, and the filled points represent the *group* average derived from the corresponding column of individual subject data points. The number of columns shown for the three groups will vary across figures, depending on the number of instances of a particular segment in the four sentences used for analysis. Because this study was descriptive in nature, no statistical comparisons across groups are reported. All necessary data required for parametric, pairwise statistical comparisons are provided for the interested reader in Appendix 4-A.

Figures 4-3 through 4-6 present data on vowel durations. For the central vowels (/ʊ/,/ʌ/,/ʊ/ [Figure 4-3]) and high-front vowels(/ɪ/, /i/ [Figure 4-4]), the Parkinson group had longer durations than both the geriatric and young adult groups. Although this difference is consistent for the three instances of central vowels and two instances of high-front vowels, the large *inter*subject variabilities associated especially with the Parkinson group, and somewhat less so with the geriatric group, indicate a need for caution in assigning meaning to the differences. The results for a diphthong and /r/-diphthong combination (/āɪ/,/rāɪ/ [Figure 4-5]) and for low-back vowels and an /r/-low-back vowel combination

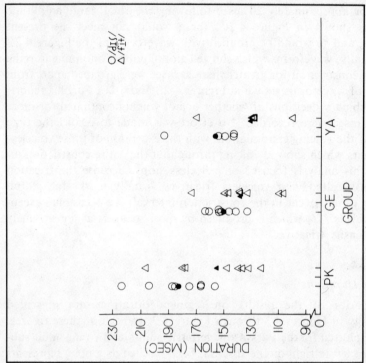

Figure 4-4   Group and individual subject mean durations for vowels /ɪ/,/iː/.

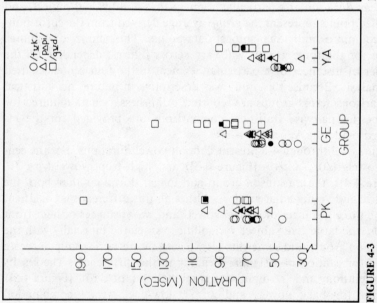

FIGURE 4-3   Group and individual subject mean durations for vowels /ʊ/, /ʌ/, /uː/.

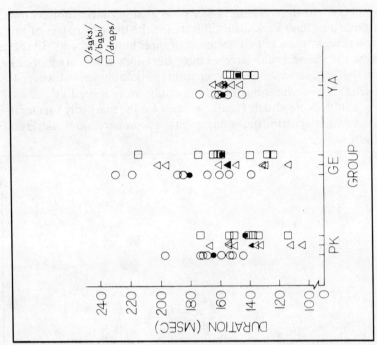

FIGURE 4-6
Group and individual subject mean durations for vowels /ɑ/, /a/, and /rɑ/ combination.

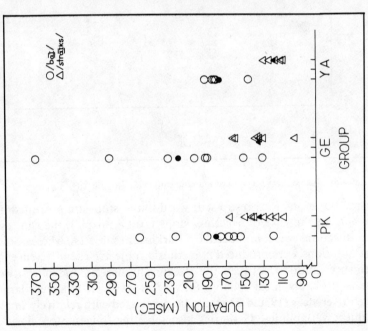

FIGURE 4-5
Group and individual subject mean durations for diphthong /āɪ/ and /r/-diphthong combination /rāɪ/.

(/sɑks/,/bɑbi/,/drɑps/ [Figure 4-6]), show that geriatric subjects have longer durations than Parkinson subjects for the three instances of low-back vowel segments and two instances of diphthong segments. In these contrasts, the young adults have segment durations which are more like those of the Parkinson subjects, whereas in the data shown in Figures 4-3 and 4-4, the vowel durations of young adults were more like those of geriatric adults. Note also in Figures 4-5 and 4-6 the markedly smaller intersubject variabilities for the young adults, as compared to geriatric and Parkinson subjects.

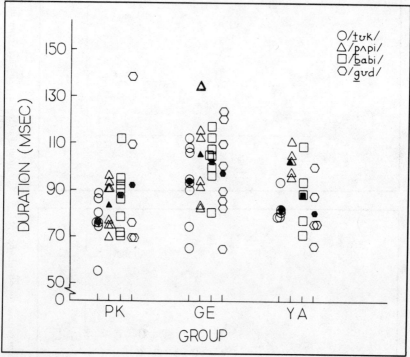

FIGURE 4-7
Group and individual subject mean durations for stops /t/, /p/, /b/, /g/.

Closure durations for prestressed, word-initial stops are presented in Figure 4-7. In the case of voiceless stops (/tʊk/, /pʌpi/), the shortest closure durations were produced by Parkinson subjects, whereas the longest durations were produced by geriatric subjects. The difference in stop closure duration between the Parkinson subjects and other two groups is probably most reliable for /p/, for which relatively large average differences (19 and 22 msec) are associated with relatively small intersubject variabilities. Geriatrics also have the longest stop closure durations for voiced stops (/b̲abi/,/g̲ʊd/), but Parkinson subjects have either the same (/b/) or longer (/g/) closure durations when compared to young adults. As in the vowel data, the Parkinson and geriatric groups are characterized by larger intersubject variabilities than the young adult group.[2]

Data on word-initial, prestressed fricative durations (/f̲it/, /s̲aks/, /s̲ʌnlaɪt/) are plotted in Figure 4-8. In each of the three instances, the Parkinson subjects have shorter fricative durations than both the geriatric and young adult subjects. These average differences, which range between 19 and 38 msec, depending on the particular group comparison and fricative, appear to be the largest and most stable effects of Parkinsonian dysarthria presented thus far. A comparison of geriatric and young adult data indicates slightly longer fricative durations for geriatric adults in /s̲aks/, a larger difference in favor of young adults for /f̲it/, and similar values for the two groups' production of /s̲ʌnlaɪt/.

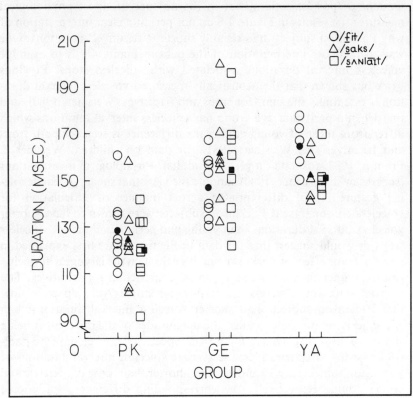

FIGURE 4-8
Group and individual subject mean durations for voiceless fricative /f/, /s/, /s/.

These data, which actually form a small subset of the data reported by Weismer and Fromm (1983), are in qualitative agreement with the full set in which young adults had longer fricative durations than geriatric adults for words in utterance-final position (i.e., like /f̱it/), but not in utterance medial position.

Actually, the labeling of the data plotted in Figure 4-8 as "fricative durations" is potentially misleading because the measurements may have included preaspiration and postaspiration (see Weismer & Elbert, 1982, p. 279). The duration measurements, which are made between the last large-amplitude glottal pulse of complex shape (see previous discussions of Data Analysis) preceding frication, and the first glottal pulse follow-ing frication, are most precisely defined as measures of the "voiceless in-terval" duration (Weismer, 1980). Usually there is only a slight dif-ference between the actual frication duration and the voiceless interval duration (approximately 12 to 20 msec, depending primarily on the amount of postaspiration), but in the absence of direct physiological measures the results in Figure 4-8 do not permit a clear interpretation of why Parkinson subjects had reliably shorter "fricative" durations. One way to facilitate interpretation of the data in Figure 4-8 is to examine voiceless interval durations associated with voiceless stops. Previous work has shown that the acoustically measured voiceless interval dura-tion is essentially the same for stops and fricatives (Weismer, 1980), and that when a particular age group has voiceless interval durations which differ from those of young adults, the difference is seen for both stops and fricatives (see Weismer, 1981, for data on children; Weismer & Fromm, 1983, for data on geriatric adults). Physiological investigations (see review in Weismer, 1980) support the view that the laryngeal devoic-ing gesture is not differentiated across manner of articulation for voiceless consonants. If Parkinson subjects were shown to have shorter voiceless interval durations than young and geriatric adults for voiceless stops, it would suggest that the data in Figure 4-8 are best explained in terms of some effect of Parkinsonian dysarthria on the laryngeal devoicing gesture, rather than on the supraglottal constriction for fricatives. The relevant data for prestressed, word-initial stops (/t̪ʊk/,/p̱ʌpi/) show that Parkinson subjects had shorter voiceless interval durations than either geriatric or young adults, the magnitudes of the differences being similar to those displayed in Figure 4-8. Specifically, when data are pool-ed across the three fricatives, the average voiceless interval durations of Parkinson subjects are 30 and 32 msec shorter than those of geriatric and young adults, respectively; the corresponding differences for pooled voiceless stops are 22 and 23 msec. Thus, the differences between Parkin-

son subjects and the other two groups shown in Figure 4-8 are probably
best understood in terms of effects on the laryngeal devoicing gesture.

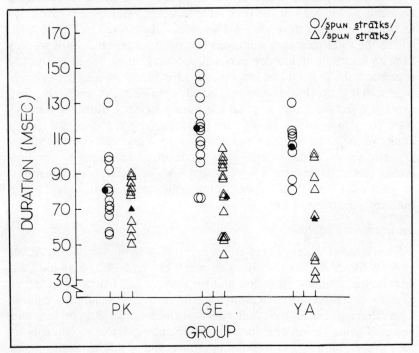

FIGURE 4-9
Group and individual subject mean durations for clustered /s/ and clustered /p/, /t/.

Figure 4-9 presents data on /s/ and stop closure durations in two
prestressed, word-initial /s/ + stop clusters (/s̲pun/ ,/st̲rāīks/).³ In this
figure, circles and triangles represent /s/ durations and stop closure
durations, respectively, and data for both clusters are plotted in the same
column. Examination of the data indicates a clear tendency for Parkinson subjects to have shorter clustered /s/ durations than either geriatric
or young adults, whereas clustered closure durations are much more
similar across groups. When the voiceless interval durations are computed for clusters, Parkinson subjects again have clearly shorter intervals
($\bar{x}$ = 184 msec) than either geriatric ($\bar{x}$ = 220 msec) or young adults ($\bar{x}$ =
225 msec). These differences are not due exclusively to the shorter
clustered /s/ durations among Parkinson subjects, as indicated by examination of the other segments (closure duration and VOT) of the
voiceless intervals.

Phrase-Level Rate

An index of phrase-level rate was obtained by summing all measured segments within each of the four sentences, and referring to these sums as "total utterance durations." These data are plotted in Figure 4-10, where the total utterance durations for the four sentences are seen to have an invariant rank order across all subject groups. When groups are compared, the shortest and longest total utterance durations were always produced by the Parkinson and geriatric subjects, respectively. The average differences across groups in total utterance duration were 45 msec for young adults versus Parkinson subjects, 75 msec for young adults versus geriatric adults and 120 msec for Parkinson subjects versus geriatric subjects. As was the case for most of the segment duration results presented in Figures 4-3 through 4-9, the intersubject variability of total utterance duration was dramatically smaller for young adults than for geriatric and Parkinson subjects.

Intrasubject Variability

Several investigators (Kent & Forner, 1980; Kent, Netsell, & Abbs, 1979; Weismer & Elbert, 1982; Weismer & Fromm, 1983) have used the intrasubject standard deviation and the derived coefficient of variation to assess precision of speech motor control for segment and phrase durations. Previous results have indicated that children, geriatric persons and persons having known or suspected neuropathologies show a tendency to have larger intrasubject variabilities than young adults. Intrasubject variability data from the present study are presented in Table 4-2, both in the form of average standard deviations for specific segments computed across subjects (first six columns of data) and average values for all segments within individual subjects (consecutive values in last column). The data points used to compute both types of average are the variances associated with repetitions of an utterance by individual subjects. The data for specific segments indicate that with the exception of one segment type (/ʊ,ʌ/), young adults always have the smallest intrasubject standard deviations, and geriatric and Parkinson subjects tend to have somewhat similar individual variabilities. Although the differences between young adults and the two older groups are consistent in several cases, the magnitude of the differences are relatively small. These subtle differences are clarified somewhat by examination of the individual subject data, which shows a certain amount of overlap between the older subject groups and the young adults. When older subjects' individual standard deviations do fall outside the young adult range, however, the values always exceed the greatest value observed for a young adult.

TABLE 4-2
Average intrasubject standard deviations reported both for selected segments pooled across subjects and for individual subjects pooled across segments.

	/a/	/aɪ/	/ii/	/ʊ,ʌ/	/t,p/	/s,f/	Individual Subject Data
Young Adults	10.26 (.064)	13.55 (.082)	11.38 (.072)	9.44 (.161)	7.27 (.074)	9.04 (.056)	9.59, 9.81, 11.02, 11.83, 12.56
Geriatrics	12.17 (.068)	21.01 (.085)	13.78 (.088)	8.56 (.121)	11.95 (.109)	13.52 (.078)	9.57, 10.46, 11.33, 11.58, 13.75, 15.49, 15.77, 19.40
Parkinson Subjects	11.67 (.063)	21.74 (.114)	15.77 (.079)	12.08 (.136)	12.78 (.136)	10.15 (.075)	10.31, 10.34, 11.48, 11.73, 14.95, 15.10, 17.48, 20.26

TABLE 4-3
Percentage of voiceless stop waveforms judged as spirantized, reported both for specific stops pooled across subjects and for individual subjects pooled across stops.

	/aɪtʌkaspunændʃf/			/ðəsʌnlɑʊtʃtɪrɑ̄ksrēīndrɑps.../				/ðənusɑks.../	/baɪbabiepʌpi/		Individual Subject Percentages
	t	k	p	t	t	k	p	k	p	p	
Young Adults	0	32	0	13	72	48	4	28	0	0	12, 14, 22, 22, 32
Geriatrics	3	20	5	5	53	44	5	38	3	10	2, 2, 8, 12, 24, 26, 26, 46
Parkinson Subjects	8	81	30	10	67	85	21	64	23	28	16, 26, 34, 42, 44, 56, 58, 61

Spirantization

Results of the spirantization analysis are reported in Table 4-3 in the form of percentages of specific stops which were judged to be spirantized. The percentage values for each stop were derived by pooling data across subjects within each group; in the right-most column of the table, individual subject percentages,rank-ordered from subjects who spirantized the fewest to most stops, are reported from data pooled across the 10 stops indicated in the table. Whereas spirantization can be seen to occur for each subject group, both the group and individual subject data indicate clearly that the phenomenon is much more typical among Parkinson subjects than among geriatric and young adults. These data also suggest that under certain conditions spirantization is not necessarily a rare phenomenon among normal speakers. For example, the three /k/s in the sentence material are spirantized a fair amount by the young adults and geriatrics, and the /t/ in /strāīks/ seems to be spirantized *typically* by young adults and about half the time by geriatric adults. It is clear, however, that those stops which have infrequent or no spirantization among normal speakers (e.g., the /p/s in the sentence material) will tend to be spirantized by persons with Parkinson's disease.

Voicing into Stop Closures

The percentages of voiceless stops for which voicing continued more than 20 msec into the closure interval are reported in Table 4-4. These group and individual subject percentages were derived in the same way as described for the spirantization analysis. Here, the data show an obvious separation between the young adults and both groups of older subjects. Young adults rarely produce voiceless stops with voicing continuing into the closure interval for more than 20 msec, whereas geriatrics and Parkinson subjects do so fairly frequently. There is a slight tendency for Parkinson subjects to produce more voiceless stops with this partial voicing criterion than geriatric subjects as suggested by a comparison of the group data, and especially the individual subject rank-ordered percentages. Although not reported in Table 4-4, there is also a slight tendency for Parkinson subjects to produce more *fully voiced* "voiceless" closures (that is, vocal fold vibration continuing through the entire closure) than geriatric subjects. This difference is mainly due to two Parkinson subjects who fully voiced approximately 45% of the "voiceless" stops. The case of the /t/ in /sʌnlāīt/ deserves special mention because of the high percentages of partially voiced closure intervals for all three groups. Perceptual analysis suggested that this sound was produced as a glottal stop by many subjects, and many of the glottal pulses which continued

TABLE 4-4
Percentage of voiceless stop waveforms judged as voiced for more than 20 msec into closure, reported for specific stops pooled across subjects and for individual subjects pooled across stops.

	/ɑ̄ɪtʌku.../		/ðəsʌnlɑ̄ɪtstrɑ̄ɪksrēindraps.../			/ðənusʌks.../	/bīɪbabɪpʌpi/		Individual Subject Percentages
	t	k	t	k	p	k	p	p	
Young Adults	16	24	52	0	4	0	24	0	10, 13, 15, 15, 20
Geriatrics	63	23	78	67	50	18	60	48	19, 25, 41, 45, 55, 63, 70, 88
Parkinson Subjects	55	58	90	51	77	63	77	49	40, 43, 50, 61, 75, 78, 79, 90

into the closure intervals appeared to be characterized by "laryngealiza-tion" (Lehiste, 1965). Priestly (1976) has presented evidence that glottal stops and laryngealization are phonetically related and often can be con-sidered as allophones of the same phoneme. It may be, therefore, that the /t/ in /sʌnlaɪt/ is not comparable to the other stops listed in Table 4-4 because of its unique phonetic status.

DISCUSSION

The purpose of this study was to provide a descriptive data base on selected articulatory characteristics of parkinsonian dysarthria. Because the study used classification variables only (that is, different subject groups), no cause and effect statements can be made about the pathophysiology of parkinsonian dysarthria. The data reported here do seem to clarify certain characteristics of this motor speech disorder, however, and may serve a heuristic function by pointing to future ex-perimental studies. Several such studies are outlined below within the context of the present findings.

Segment and Phrase-level Timing

There is a certain amount of disagreement in the literature concerning the speech timing characteristics of persons with Parkinson's disease (see review in Darley et al., 1975, pp. 190-192). The speaking rate has been perceived either as abnormally fast or slow, or as normal; more physical-ly based measures have suggested that Parkinson subjects and age-matched "normal" speakers have essentially the same speaking rate (e.g., Canter, 1963). This issue is complicated by the complex relation-ship between spatio-temporal characteristics of articulation and the perception of speaking rate (see Miller, 1981, for a review). For example, the demonstration of "normal" syllable durations, total utterance dura-tions, words per minute, or any physical measure of speaking time may not be associated with a rate that is perceived as "normal." Kent and Rosenbek (1982) have suggested that certain persons with Parkinson's disease may have "normal" speech timing, but be perceived as having abnormally fast rates because they blur certain acoustic contrasts which are normally quite prominent in the speech wave. The blurred contrasts result from faulty spatial or spatio-temporal adjustments of the ar-ticulators, such as is thought to be the problem in spirantization of stops.

The present data suggest the Parkinsonian dysarthria may be characterized by some subtle reductions in segment durations and total utterance durations relative to older "normal" speakers. Parkinson sub-jects had, on average, shorter segment durations than geriatric subjects for two vowel groups (/aɪ/,/a/), as well as stops and fricatives. Parkinson subjects also had consistently shorter total utterance durations than geriatric subjects. Only in the case of the high-front vowel group (/i/, /ɪ/) and the mid-vowels (/ʊ/,/ʌ/,/ʌ/), did the Parkinson subjects have longer vowel durations than geriatric subjects. The tendency for geriatrics to have the longest segment and phrase-level durations is probably not surprising, both because aging has often been associated with slowing of both cognitive and neuromuscular performance (Gutmann & Hanzlikova, 1975; Surwillo, 1968) and some studies of speech timing (Benjamin, 1982; Mysak, 1959) have shown geriatric adults to have slightly longer phrase and segment durations than young adults. What is more interesting in the present data are the frequent similarities in speech timing — especially for total utterance durations — for Parkinson subjects and young adults. One might expect the segment and phrase durations of Parkinson subjects to be more similar to those of geriatric subjects rather than young adults, because the Parkinson subjects are approaching or in the geriatric age range. This may imply that Parkinsonian dysarthria is often characterized by a slightly accelerated speaking rate relative to the speech production behavior of the *appropriate comparison group* (that is, geriatric people).

In the well known Mayo Clinic study (Darley et al., 1969a, 1969b), parkinsonian dysarthrics were unique among dysarthrics in being perceived as having a slightly faster than average speaking rate. The present data seem to provide some objective support for these judgments, but the question may be asked — Why would parkinsonian speech be perceived as slightly fast if the timing characteristics are often like those of "normal" young adults? Part of the answer may be found in the "blurred contrast" hypothesis proposed by Kent and Rosenbek (1982) (see also Netsell, Daniel, & Celesia, 1975), and part may be related to a flexible expectation of what an "average" speaking rate should be, based on perceived speaker age. Parkinson subjects tend to have gerontological voice characteristics such as high fundamental frequency (f_o) (Canter, 1963) and vocal roughness (see Darley et al., 1975; Schley, Fenton, & Niimi, 1982) that may be somewhat exaggerated relative to an individual subject's chronological age. Listeners may associate such voice characteristics with older individuals and, therefore, slower speaking rates; thus, the combination of gerontological voice characteristics paired with young adult speaking rates may be perceived as speech produced with faster than (gerontological) average speaking rates. Both the "blurred contrast" and "speaking rate expectation" hypotheses could be evaluated using synthetic speech material. For example, listeners might be asked to scale the rate of utterances which are manipulated for voice characteristics only, or for distinctiveness of acoustic contrasts.

The "speaking rate expectation" hypothesis predicts that utterances with identical timing characteristics should be judged as having faster rates as the source parameters are adjusted in the direction of gerontological characteristics. The "blurred contrast" hypothesis predicts that utterances with identical timing characteristics should be judged as having faster rates as acoustic discontinuities in the speech wave are eliminated or replaced by more continuous waveform features. The clinical impact of such studies might be that positive findings in either or both of the above experiments would argue against a primary rehabilitative focus on speaking rate in certain cases of Parkinson's disease.

The Voiceless Interval
and Voicing of Voiceless Stops

The greatest group difference for segment duration was found for the voiceless interval. The Parkinson subjects produced voiceless interval durations for fricatives, stops, and /s/ + stop clusters that were substantially and consistently shorter than the voiceless interval durations of geriatrics and young adults. Weismer and Fromm (1983) speculated that the shorter voiceless interval durations they observed for geriatric adults, as compared to young adults, could be explained by known age-related changes in laryngeal muscles and other tissues which tend to stiffen the movable structures. If this increased stiffness reduced the lateral excursion of the vocal folds associated with the laryngeal devoicing gesture, it would contribute to the shortening of the voiceless interval.

Parkinson subjects may have even shorter voiceless interval durations than geriatric subjects because of exaggerated deterioration of laryngeal tissues, disordered central drive to the posterior cricoarytenoid muscle, or an interaction of the former and latter. In a recent study of electromyographic and movement patterns associated with walking, Dietz, Quintern, and Berger (1981) demonstrated that muscular rigidity in Parkinson's disease could not be explained on the basis of disordered central drive. These authors concluded that atrophy of muscle fibers, and perhaps specifically of fibers making up phasic motor units, must be responsible for the observed muscular rigidity. If similar changes occur throughout the laryngeal muscles or in the posterior cricoarytenoid muscle specifically, the resulting muscular rigidity would probably reduce contractile efficiency of the posterior cricoarytenoid muscle, thus shortening the time course of the laryngeal devoicing gesture (that is, the voiceless interval). Histological studies on parkinsonian larynges are needed to determine if muscle fibers show greater deterioration than would be predicted by chronological age or if muscle fibers are uniquely affected by the disease state.

It is also probable that some component of the reduced voiceless interval duration is related to dysfunction of laryngeal central drive. Plasse and Lieberman (1981) have reviewed evidence that general deterioration in Parkinson's disease may be accompanied by progressive laryngeal deterioration toward an endpoint of laryngeal paralysis. A diminished central drive to the posterior cricoarytenoid muscle might weaken the laryngeal devoicing gesture to the point where only a very small glottal maximum would be reached, thus allowing voicing to begin soon after the onset of the gesture. The combination of muscular deterioration with diminished or disordered central drive to the larynx no doubt accounts for the short voiceless intervals, high f_o, and rough voice quality of parkinsonian speech. It would be interesting to study changes in these three variables as individual cases of parkinsonism progress, because a progressive and general laryngeal deterioration would seem to predict that change in these variables should co-occur.

One finding of the present study which indicates that the deterioration of laryngeal function in parkinsonian speech is partly explainable as a normal aging process is the similar tendency of geriatric and Parkinson subjects to continue vocal fold vibration into closure intervals of phonologically voiceless stops. If the data reported in Table 4-4 are accurate, continued voicing of voiceless stops should not be considered a unique feature of parkinsonian dysarthria, except in the case of isolated patients who fully voice "voiceless" closures. Perhaps the continuation of voicing observed for subjects in both older groups reflects the difficulty of initiating the laryngeal devoicing gesture because of stiffened laryngeal structures and/or diminished central drive.

Spirantization

The present data suggest that *frequent* spirantization of stops is a unique characteristic of parkinsonian dysarthria (see also Kent & Netsell, 1979). Spirantization also occurs occasionally among both young and old normal speakers, especially in the case of dorsal stops. In fact, cinefluorographic observations (Kent & Moll, 1972) suggest that dorsal stops may be produced by a sliding motion of the tongue dorsum along the soft and hard palates, this motion often being characterized by an incomplete (i.e., leaking) lingual-palatal constriction. Moreover, cluster analyses of consonant confusions in syllable-memory experiments (Klatt, 1968; Weismer, 1975) have demonstrated an affinity of dorsal stops for *fricative* categories. Thus, the current finding of relatively frequent spirantization of /k/ by normal speakers is not necessarily surprising;

more data should be obtained on patterns of spirantization for dorsal stops in word-initial position,as all /k/s in the current analysis occurred only as word-final singletons or in word-final clusters.

Why should Parkinson subjects spirantize stops more often than normal speakers? A reduced range of articulator movement, either due to acceleration (Netsell et al., 1975; see also Hirose et al., 1982; Hirose et al., 1981) or rigidity resulting from agonist-antagonist co-contraction (Hunker et al., 1982) could explain the phenomenon. It would be interesting to know if an index of acceleration or rigidity would predict individual spirantization patterns among a group of Parkinson subjects. For example, Hunker et al. (1982) reported an inverse relationship between degree of lip stiffness and amount of lip displacement during articulatory sequences. This finding would be quite compelling — at least with respect to diagnostic and prognostic considerations in speech pathology — if it could be shown that measurement of articulator stiffness or displacement predicts frequency of spirantization.[4] If this were the case, the less costly and more efficient acoustic measures could be used to make direct inferences about the status of aticulatory musculature in Parkinson subjects. Because Hunker et al. (1982) did not report phonetic or acoustic data, it is impossible to determine what their data mean in terms of the speech pathology associated with Parkinson's disease.

Variability

It has been noted previously (Kent & Netsell, 1979) that Parkinsonian dysarthria, like other dysarthrias, is a heterogeneous phenomenon. A comparison across groups of the intersubject variabilities displayed in Figures 4-3 through 4-10 suggests that this heterogeneity may be more characteristic of agedness in general than Parkinson's disease in particular. Greater variability among geriatric as compared to young adult populations on almost any biological or behavioral measure is an often observed phenomenon, typically attributed to different rates of aging within a group of aged cohorts (Birren & Renner, 1977).

A similar conclusion seems appropriate for the findings of intrasubject variability (Table 4-2). On the average, both geriatrics and Parkinson subjects had individual standard deviations for segment durations which were slightly greater than those of young adults. In addition, inspection of the average intrasubject standard deviations on a subject-by-subject basis shows some overlap between members of the older groups and of the young adult group; when subjects in either of the older groups fall outside the young adult range, however, the values are typically greater than the largest young adult value. This suggests that certain geriatric

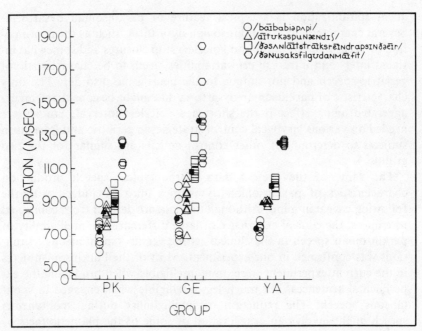

FIGURE 4-10
Group and individual subject mean durations for total utterance durations of four sentences.

speakers may show a tendency to lose some control of the temporal structure of articulatory sequences. Because the largest performance differences between geriatric and young adults tend to emerge under conditions which induce biological or cognitive stress (Ordy, 1975; Surwillo, 1968), it would be interesting to obtain intrasubject variabilities for segment durations produced when the speech mechanism is placed under some form of performance stress. For example, data derived from the fast speaking rate condition (see *Methods* earlier in chapter) may show more clearly the differences in the stability of speech timing (see Weismer & Fromm, 1983) between normal geriatric and young adults, and perhaps between normal geriatric and Parkinson subjects. Based on the current data, however, the timing stability characteristics of Parkinsonian dysarthria would appear to be "normal."

CONCLUSIONS AND A CAVEAT

The data presented here suggest that Parkinson subjects have segmental and phrase-level durations which are slightly shorter than the corresponding durations of the appropriate control group, and that frequent spirantization is a typical feature of parkinsonian dysarthria. Several characteristics of parkinsonian dysarthria, such as the continuation of vocal fold vibration into voiceless stop closures and somewhat inflated inter- and intra-subject variabilities, seem to be characteristic of geriatric speech and not unique to the neurogenic disorder. The only characteristic of parkinsonian dysarthria that might be considered an exaggerated aging effect is the shortened voiceless interval. Studies are needed on various laryngeal control strategies in geriatric and Parkinson subjects to determine if other control deficits are similar for the two groups.

The value of the present data to the typical speech production characteristics of parkinsonian dysarthrics must be judged with the following caveat in mind. Although the data are derived from connected utterances, the clinical experience of large differences in intelligibility of parkinsonian speech in the clinical setting versus "spontaneous" situations was confirmed in our experiment. Most of the Parkinson subjects in the current experiment were quite intelligible when producing the experimental sentences, but much less intelligible when engaged in spontaneous speech. The reduction of intelligibility during spontaneous speech might involve an exaggeration of some of the phonetic facts of parkinsonian dysarthria described in this chapter, but our impression is that differences between the two forms of speech are much more complex than simply faster rate, more spirantization, and so forth. Careful acoustic and physiological analyses of the spontaneous speech of a few subjects would be quite valuable in understanding how to bridge the gap between the clinical and ecological manifestations of parkinsonian dysarthria.

NOTES

[1]Vowel durations were measured from the first to last large-amplitude, complex-shape glottal pulse associated with an open vocal tract event. When vowels followed voiceless stops, therefore, these durations did not include the VOT. Fricative durations were measured from the final large-amplitude, complex-shape glottal pulse preceding aperiodic energy to the first glottal pulse following the aperiodic waveform; this measurement also corresponds to the *voiceless interval duration,* which is discussed further in the Results section. Voiced and voiceless stop durations were measured from the final large-amplitude, complex-shape glottal pulse preceding either a "silent" interval or an interval containing low amplitude, simple-shape glottal pulses, to the burst associated with release of the supraglottal constriction. /s/ durations in /s/ + stop clusters were measured from the final large-amplitude, complex-shape glottal pulse preceding aperiodic energy to the reduction of this aperiodicity to baseline; stop durations in the same clusters were measured from the

latter point to the stop burst. Voice-onset times, which are not reported on directly in this chapter (but are a component of the voiceless interval for voiceless stops) were measured from the stop burst to the first following glottal pulse.

[2]When closure durations for stops in poststressed position are examined (that is, /drɑps/, /baḇi/,/pʌp̱i/), there appears to be little or no difference between the groups. This indicates that the group differences observed in Figure 4-7 must be qualified by position-in-word and/or stress effects. Poststressed consonant durations are known to be less affected than prestressed consonant durations by phonetic conditioning factors (Ingrisano & Weismer, 1979; Klatt, 1974), and it is possible that group differences in speech timing are also less likely to be observed in the vicinity of secondary and lesser stress. This hypothesis should be tested carefully because of the implications for both remediation of speech disorders and theories of speech production.

[3]The voiceless interval for /s/ + stop clusters includes the events between the last glottal pulse preceding the fricative, and the first glottal pulse following the stop burst. In a segmental terminology, it includes the fricative, stop closure, and voice-onset time.

[4]"Frequency of spirantization" is only used as an example here, as the potential for other predictive relationships (such as between articulator stiffness and centralization of vowels) should be studied.

REFERENCES

Appel, S. H. A unifying hypothesis for the cause of amyotrophic lateral scelerosis, parkinsonism, and alzheimer disease. *Annals of Neurology,* 1981, *10,* 499-505.

Benjamin, B. J. Phonological performance in gerontological speech. *Journal of Psycholinguistic Research,* 1982, *11,* 159-167.

Birren, J. E., & Renner, V. J. Research on the psychology of aging: Principles and experimentation. In J. E. Birren & K. W. Schaie (Eds.), *Handbook of the psychology of aging.* New York: Van Nostrand Reinhold, 1977, 3-38.

Canter, G. J. Speech characteristics of patients with Parkinson's disease: I. Intensity, pitch, and duration. *Journal of Speech and Hearing Disorders,* 1963, *28,* 221-229.

Canter, G. J. Speech characteristics of patients with Parkinson's disease: III. Articulation, diadochokinesis, and overall speech adequacy. *Journal of Speech and Hearing Disorders,* 1965, *30,* 217-224.

Critchley, E. M. R. Speech disorders of parkinsonian: a review. *Journal of Neurology, Neurosurgery, and Psychiatry,* 1981, *44,* 751-758.

Darley, F. L., Aronson, A. E., & Brown, J. R. Differential diagnostic patterns of dysarthria. *Journal of Speech and Hearing Research,* 1969, *12,* 246-269. (a)

Darley, F. L., Aronson, A. E., & Brown, J. R. Clusters of deviant speech dimensions in the dysarthrias. *Journal of Speech and Hearing Research,* 1969, *12,* 462-496. (b)

Darley, F. L., Aronson, A. E., & Brown, J. R. *Motor speech disorders.* Philadelphia: Saunders, 1975.

DeLong, M., & Georgopoulos, A. P. Motor functions of the basal ganglia. In V. B. Brooks (Ed.), *Handbook of physiology,* Section 1 (Vol. 2: Motor control, Part 2). Bethesda, MD: American Physiological Society, 1981, 1017-1061.

Dietz, V., Quintern, J., & Berger, W. Electrophysiological studies of gait in spasticity and rigidity: Evidence that altered mechanical properties of muscle contribute to hypertonia. *Brain,* 1981, *104,* 431-449.

Gutmann, E., & Hanzlikova, V. Changes in neuromuscular relationships in aging. In J. M. Ordy & K. R. Brizzee (Eds.), *Neurobiology of aging.* New York: Plenum Press, 1975, 193-207.

Hirose, H., Kiritani, S., & Sawashima, M. Velocity of articulatory movements in normal and dysarthric subjects. *Folia Phoniatrica,* 1982, *34,* 210-215.

Hirose, H., Kiritani, S., Ushijima, T., Yoshioka, H., & Sawashima, M. Patterns of dysarthric movements in patients with Parkinsonism. *Folia Phoniatrica,* 1981, *33,* 204-215.

Hunker, C. J., Abbs, J. H., & Barlow, S. M. The relationship between parkinsonian rigidity and hypokinesia in the orofacial system: A quantitative analysis. *Neurology,* 1982, *32*(7), 749-754.

Ingrisano, D., & Weismer, G. /s/ duration: Methodological influences and linguistic variables. *Phonetica,* 1979, *36,* 32-43.

Kent, R. D., & Forner, L. L. Speech segment durations in sentence recitations by children and adults. *Journal of Phonetics,* 1980, *8,* 157-168.

Kent, R. D., & Moll, K. L. Cinefluorographic analyses of selected lingual consonants. *Journal of Speech and Hearing Research,* 1972, *15,* 453-473.

Kent, R. D., & Netsell, R. *Acoustic-phonetic features of Parkinsonian dysarthria.* Paper presented at the annual convention of the American Speech and Hearing Association, Atlanta, 1979.

Kent, R. D., Netsell, R. & Abbs, J. H. Acoustic characteristics of dysarthria associated with cerebellar disease. *Journal of Speech and Hearing Research,* 1979, *22,* 627-648.

Kent, R. D., & Rosenbek, J. C. Prosodic disturbances and neurologic lesion. *Brain and Language,* 1982, *15,* 259-291.

Kent, R. D. & Rosenbek, J. C. Acoustic patterns of apraxia of speech. *Journal of Speech and Hearing Research,* 1983, *26,* 231-249.

Klatt, D. H. Structure of confusions in short-term memory between English consonants. *Journal of the Acoustical Society of America,* 1968, *44,* 401-407.

Klatt, D. H. The duration of [s] in English words. *Journal of Speech and Hearing Research,* 1974, *17,* 51-63.

Leanderson, R., Persson, A., & Öhman, S. Electromyographic studies of the function of the facial muscles in dysarthria. *Acta Otolaryngologica Supplementum,* 1970, *263,* 89-94.

Lehiste, I. Some acoustic characteristics of dysarthric speech. *Bibliotheca Phonetica,* Fasc. 2. Basel: Karger, 1965.

Logemann, J. A., & Fisher, H. B. Vocal tract control in Parkinson's disease: Phonetic feature analysis of misarticulation. *Journal of Speech and Hearing Disorders,* 1981, *46,* 348-352.

McGeer, E., & McGeer, P. Age changes in the human for some enzymes associated with metabolism of colecholamines, GABA, and acetylcholine. In J. Ordy & I. Brizzee (Ed.), *Neurobiology of aging.* New York: Plenum Press, 1975.

Miller, J. L. Effects of speaking rate on segmental distinctions. In P. D. Eimas & J. L. Miller (Eds.), *Perspectives on the study of speech.* Hillsdale, NJ: Lawrence Erlbaum, 1981, 39-74.

Mysak, E. D. Pitch and duration characteristics of older males. *Journal of Speech and Hearing Research,* 1959, *2,* 46-54.

Netsell, R., Daniel, B., & Celesia, G. G. Acceleration and weakness in Parkinsonian dysarthria. *Journal of Speech and Hearing Disorders,* 1975, *40,* 170-178.

Ordy, J. M. The nervous system, behavior, and aging: An interdisciplinary lifespan approach. In J. M. Ordy & K. R. Brizzee (Eds.), *Neurobiology of aging.* New York: Plenum Press, 1975, 85-118.

Petajan, J., & Jarcho, L. Motor unit control in Parkinson's disease and the influence of levodopa. *Neurology,* 1975, *25,* 866-869.

Plasse, H. M., & Lieberman, A. N. Bilateral vocal cord paralysis in Parkinson's disease. *Archives of Otolaryngology,* 1981, *107,* 252-253.

Priestly, T. M. S. A note on the glottal stop. *Phonetica,* 1976, *33,* 268-274.

Schley, W. S., Fenton, E., & Niimi, S. Vocal symptoms in Parkinson's disease treated with levodopa: A case report. *Annals of Otology, Rhinology and Laryngology,* 1982, *91,* 119-121.

Semjen, A. From motor learning to sensorimotor skill acquisition. *Journal of Human Movement Studies,* 1977, *3,* 182-191.

Surwillo, W. W. Timing of behavior in senescence and the role of the central nervous system. In G. A. Talland (Ed.), *Human aging and behavior: Recent advances in research and theory.* New York: Academic Press, 1968, 1-35.

Weismer, G. *Consonant intrusion errors in auditory and visual short-term memory.* Unpublished doctoral dissertation, University of Wisconsin — Madison, 1975.

Weismer, G. Control of the voicing distinction for intervocalic stops and fricatives: Some data and theoretical considerations. *Journal of Phonetics,* 1980, *8,* 417-428.

Weismer, G. *Temporal characteristics of the laryngeal devoicing gesture for voiceless consonants and fricative-stop clusters: Influences of vowel environment and speaker age.* Paper presented at the 101st meeting of the Acoustical Society of America, Ottowa, Ontario, 1981.

Weismer, G., Dinnsen, D., & Elbert, M. A study of the voicing distinction associated with omitted, word-final stops. *Journal of Speech and Hearing Disorders,* 1981, *46,* 320-327.

Weismer, G., & Elbert, M. Temporal characteristics of "functionally"-misarticulated /s/ in four- to six-year old children. *Journal of Speech and Hearing Research,* 1982, *25,* 275-287.

Weismer, G., & Fromm, D. Acoustic analysis of geriatric utterances: Segmental and nonsegmental characteristics which relate to laryngeal function. In D. M. Bless & J. H. Abbs (Eds.), *Vocal fold physiology.* San Diego: College-Hill Press, 1983.

ACKNOWLEDGMENT

This work was supported by NS 13274-05. Davida Fromm, Cynthia Chicouris, and Beth Ansel assisted with processing of subjects and preparation of graphics. Special thanks are due to Edie Swift for locating the Parkinson and geriatric subjects.

APPENDIX

Data displayed in Figures 3–10 of text. Numbers displayed as: Mean (intersubject standard deviation) (*N* of subjects contributing to mean and *SD*). Data pooled across segment types are just below each group of individual segment values. Missing data are usually associated with blurred contrasts that precluded measurement.

	Parkinson subjects	Geriatrics	Young adults
tʊk	66 (11) (7)	53 (11) (8)	45 (4) (5)
gʊd	101 (44) (5)	89 (23) (8)	73 (12) (5)
pʌpi	74 (14) (8)	65 (10) (8)	54 (13) (5)
/ʊ,ʊ,ʌ/	78 (28) (20)	69 (22) (24)	57 (15) (15)
/dɪʃ	183 (21) (8)	150 (9) (8)	156 (19) (5)
fɪt	155 (27) (8)	137 (20) (8)	131 (22) (5)
/ɪ,i/	173 (34) (16)	144 (17) (16)	144 (24) (10)
baɪ	181 (41) (8)	220 (72) (8)	177 (16) (5)
straɪks	134 (17) (8)	136 (19) (8)	118 (8) (5)
/aɪ, raɪ/	158 (39) (16)	178 (67) (16)	147 (32) (10)
bab	139 (20) (8)	155 (30) (8)	156 (6) (5)
saks	165 (16) (8)	181 (30) (8)	159 (9) (5)
draps	143 (17) (7)	159 (27) (8)	147 (7) (5)
/a,a,ra/	149 (21) (23)	165 (31) (24)	154 (9) (15)
tʊk	76 (10) (7)	93 (15) (8)	82 (6) (5)
pʌpi	83 (10) (8)	105 (20) (8)	102 (5) (5)
/t,p/	80 (10) (15)	99 (19) (16)	92 (11) (10)
babi	87 (13) (8)	102 (11) (8)	87 (13) (5)
gʊd	92 (27) (5)	97 (19) (8)	80 (11) (5)
/b,g/	89 (20) (13)	99 (16) (16)	84 (13) (10)
sʌnlaɪt	120 (15) (8)	154 (23) (8)	151 (9) (5)
sacks	124 (16) (8)	162 (20) (8)	152 (10) (5)
fɪt	128 (15) (8)	147 (12) (8)	164 (9) (5)
/s,s,f/	124 (16) (24)	154 (20) (24)	156 (11) (15)
/sp,st/	81 (20) (12)	116 (23) (15)	105 (15) (8)
/sp,st/	70 (16) (11)	76 (20) (15)	64 (27) (9)
TUD			
Buy Bobby...	716 (90) (8)	798 (106) (8)	733 (34) (5)
I took a spoon...	834 (66) (7)	901 (101) (8)	888 (13) (5)
The sunlight...	894 (62) (7)	1079 (112) (8)	993 (34) (5)
The new socks...	1247 (143) (7)	1391 (230) (8)	1256 (14) (5)

5

Assessment of Stress Patterning

Kathryn M. Yorkston
David R. Beukelman
Fred D. Minifie
Shimon Sapir

INTRODUCTION

The ability of a speaker to stress accurately important words and syllables in an utterance is critical in human communication. Stress patterning allows the speaker to mark specific locations within an utterance where the listener can decode significant semantic and syntactic information, thereby improving the efficiency of communication. Usually this is done through an alternative stress pattern in which content words (nouns, pronouns, adjectives, adverbs, and verbs) are produced with greater prominence than are function words (prepositions, articles, and connectives, Lehiste, 1970). Normal stress patterning is less well understood by the scientific community than are most other aspects of human communication. Further, despite the nearly universal presence of stress deficits in dysarthric speakers, only recently have these deficits begun to be described in the scientific literature (Barnes, 1983; Kent & Rosenbek, 1982) or addressed in treatment (Caligiuri & Murry, 1983;

Murry, 1983; Rosenbek & LaPointe, 1978; Simmons, 1983). From a clinical perspective, optimizing stress patterning in a dysarthric speaker is essential because such patterns enhance the transfer of meaning from speaker to listener, reduce monotony, improve the intelligibility, and contribute to the naturalness of speech.

For purposes of the present chapter, stress will be considered both a linguistic and perceptual term, referring to the level of prominence of a syllable within an utterance (Chomsky & Halle, 1968; Lehiste, 1970). Syllable prominence appears to be signaled by the interaction of several suprasegmental acoustic parameters, including voice fundamental frequency, voice intensity, and the durational patterning of syllables (Lea, Medress, & Skinner, 1972). The basic role of these variables in coding syllable prominence is generally acknowledged. Stressed syllables usually have higher fundamental frequencies and voice intensities than do unstressed syllables, and stressed syllables are usually longer in duration than unstressed syllables. However, the frequency of occurrence of counter-examples to these general rules gives an indication of the complexity of finding simple acoustic correlates to perceived stress. For example, certain acoustic parameters serve other functions in addition to signaling prominence. Fundamental frequency shifts and syllable lengthening may serve as boundary features. In many instances, an unstressed syllable in the final position of a sentence may be longer than stressed syllables occurring elsewhere within the utterance. Thus, the significance of each of the main stress cues (frequency, intensity, and syllable duration) appears to vary from one location to another within an utterance (Cheung, Holden, & Minifie, 1973.)

Lieberman (1960) describes "trading effects" among the main stress cues in which lack of differentiation in one acoustic parameter may be offset by pronounced changes in another. Although the interaction among the main stress cues is essential for the understanding of stress patterning, much research has been directed at the influence of a single acoustic parameter on the stress level of a single syllable. For example, Bleakley (1973), Atkinson (1976), and O'Shaughnessy (1979) studied the role of fundamental frequency in coding stress. Fry (1955) studied duration and intensity as cues to stress. Chueng, et al. (1973) looked at several acoustic parameters as individual and collective features. Most investigators agree that some attribute of the fundamental frequency domain is a strong signaler of stress during normal speech production (Morton & Jassem, 1965), but that the other acoustic variables also contribute to the magnitude of stress applied to a syllable. For example, the infrastructure of prosodic patterning, changes in fundamental frequency

(ΔF) and intensity (ΔI) within a syllable, are known to influence perceptual judgments of stress.

While knowledge of normal stress patterning is incomplete, our understanding of stress patterning by dysarthric speakers is further complicated by disruptions in the motor control of speech production. Physiologically, "extra effort" is required during production of a prominent syllable, in comparison to the effort required during production of the same syllable in an unstressed position (Ohman, 1967; Netsell, 1973). When dysarthric speakers attempt to produce increased physiologic effort in the presence of neuromotor impairment of the speech mechanism, stress patterning may be inaccurate, exaggerated, or in other ways bizarre.

Although researchers are beginning to document prosodic disruptions in dysarthric speech, clinicians have few tools with which to approach the evaluation and treatment of abnormalities of stress patterning in their clients. Darley, Aronson, and Brown (1969a, 1969b, 1975) reported a perceptual scaling approach for evaluating 38 speech dimensions including several aspects of prosody — reduced stress, excess and equal stress, monopitch, and monoloudness. Rosenbek and LaPointe (1978) suggested that contrastive stress sentences were useful in the evaluation and treatment of stressing anomalies in the dysarthric population; however, no specific measurement techniques were provided.

Because stress prominence is a perceptual phenomenon, the quantification of stressing anomalies should have at its core perceptual judgments. In the analysis of dysarthric speakers' stress patterning the two most relevant perceptual judgments appear to be the accuracy of the stress patterning and the bizarreness of the application of the acoustic cues used to signal stress. The purpose of this chapter is threefold. First, the accuracy and bizarreness of the stress patterning of three mildly dysarthric speakers are perceptually determined. Second, selected acoustic parameters for coding stress by these dysarthric speakers — peak fundamental frequency, syllable duration, and relative syllable intensity — are analyzed, described, and compared to normal speakers. Third, the implications of this illustrative data are discussed in terms of clinical assessment and treatment of dysarthric speakers with prosodic disturbances.

METHODS AND PROCEDURES

Selection of Speakers

Data selected to illustrate stress patterning for this chapter came from a larger study of dysarthric speakers. The larger study compares utterances produced by groups of dysarthric speakers who vary in type and severity with those of a group of normal speakers. Three dysarthric speakers were selected for this report. These three speakers were all identified as having predominantly ataxic dysarthria, and all were judged as mildly dysarthric with sentence intelligibility scores over 95 percent as measured on The Assessment of Intelligibility of Dysarthric Speech developed by Yorkston and Beukelman (1981). The dysarthric speakers were selected because they were similar in type and overall severity. A more detailed description of each dysarthric speaker appears in the Results section.

Twenty normal native speakers of American English (10 males and 10 females) participated as a control group for this study. None of the normal speakers had a history of speech, language, hearing, or neurological disorders. They ranged in age from 19 to 44 years of age.

Speech Sample and Audio Recording Procedures

From a larger sample of 10 stimulus sentences, 3 were selected for the present anlaysis. These sentences were produced by varying the stress location within the sentence, *Show Sam some snow.* The resulting stimulus sentences and antecedent comments are listed in Table 5-1. The sentence *Show Sam some snow* was selected for this preliminary analysis

Table 5-1
Shown below are the sentences analyzed in this study—all are variations of the sentences *Show Sam some snow.* Variations were produced by shifting the locations of linguistic stress in the sentence in response to the examiner's antecedent comments. The syllable receiving primary stress is shown in dark type.

Examiner's Comment:	Speakers' Response:
To whom should I show the snow?	Show **Sam** some snow.
Should I show Sam all the snow?	Show Sam **some** snow.
What should I show Sam?	Show Sam some **snow**.

because it was characterized by a number of features which simplified data analysis. It contained only single-syllable words and a simple falling fundamental frequency pattern. All of the dysarthric and normal speakers correctly identified the locus of intended stress for the three different stressing patterns of the sentence with targeted stress on the words — *Sam, some,* and *snow,* respectively. Although the stimulus sentences for this experiment initially may seem artificial, they were constructed to meet two criteria: (1) that the pattern of adjacent phonemes would permit durational segmentation from a raw acoustic wave form, and (2) that normal speakers were consistently able to produce targeted stress.

Simultaneous audio recordings of speaker performance were made on a TEAC stereo recorder (Model: A-2300SX) from a contact neck microphone positioned over the lateral aspect of the thyroid cartilage of the larynx and an airborne microphone positioned 6 inches anterior to the lips. All recordings were made in a sound-treated room.

Each stimulus sentence was printed on a separate sheet of paper. Each speaker was instructed to produce the stimulus sentence in response to an antecedent comment by the examiner. The examiner's antecedent comment was designed to facilitate the speaker's production of a specific stress pattern. For example, if the examiner's antecedent comment was "Should I show Sam all the snow?" the speaker's correct response would be *Show Sam - some - snow*, with the primary stress produced on the word *some*. Speakers were audio recorded, as they produced all stimulus sentences two times.

Following each sentence production, the speaker was asked to identify the word that he or she had intended to make the most prominent. In this way, the speaker's understanding of the task was confirmed. Without exception, normal speakers were able to identify the appropriate syllable targeted for stress. Dysarthric speakers identified the appropriate stress targets 97% of the time. When a speaker did not correctly identify the syllable targeted for stress, that utterance was excluded from further analysis.

Perceptual Analysis of Stress

A master tape containing only the speakers' utterances and not the antecedent comments produced by the examiner to elicit the desired stress patterning was constructed for use during the perceptual rating of stress patterning. Thus, the tape could be judged without knowledge of the intended locus of primary stress. The relative level of perceived stress for each syllable was rated according to a system developed by Chueng et al.(1973). Three judges rated the relative stress of each syllable by placing a mark on a continuous scale similar to the one illustrated in Figure 5-1, which contains an example of a judge's rating of a sentence where *Sam* is the syllable targeted for stress. The top of the scale denoted "most possible" stress and the bottom denoted "least possible" stress. The scaling marks were quantified by measuring the location of the mark on the scale. Prior to judging the master tape, each judge was trained in the use of the rating system until a criterion level of 90% accuracy on location of primary stress was reached while rating the overall stress pattern of

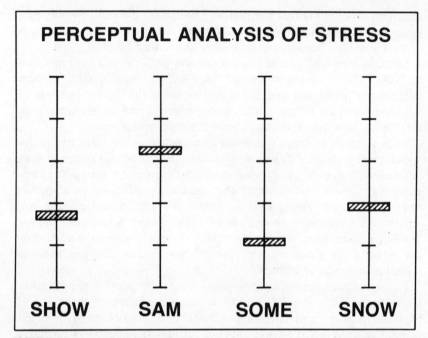

FIGURE 5-1
A judge's estimates of the prominence of each syllable of a sentence in which *Sam* is targeted for primary stress. The top of the scale denotes "most possible" stress and the bottom denotes "least possible" stress.

sentences produced by 10 speakers (dysarthric and normal) whose samples were not included on the master tape.

As a result of the analysis of perceived stress, the investigators were able to determine whether an utterance was (1) appropriately stressed with all judges in agreement that the locus of perceived stress was on the targeted syllable, (2) inappropriately stressed with all judges in agreement that the locus of stress was not on the targeted syllable, or (3) perceptually confusing with the judges in disagreement about the locus of the stress.

Perceptual Judgments of Bizarreness

A pilot study for this project demonstrated that shifts in acoustic parameters which are used to signal stress patterning also are perceived along a speech dimension which ranges from *natural* to *bizarre*. Therefore, it became apparent that at least a gross indication of degree of bizarreness was necessary in order to interpret the acoustic data. Judges were given a series of audio cassettes each containing all of the sentences produced by the three dysarthric speakers and those of one normal male speaker. Judges were instructed to listen to all the cassettes and rank order them from least bizarre to most bizarre. Speech bizarreness was defined as a marked deviation from a natural production. Bizarre speech was defined as deviating from an expected pattern or as unconventional in terms of intonation, voice quality, rate, rhythm, or intensity adjustments. Judges were instructed that bizarreness was not to be considered synonymous with unintelligibility, nor was bizarreness to be considered an index to severity of dysarthria. Thus it was possible for a mildly dysarthric individual to be judged as very bizarre and for a severely dysarthric speaker to be perceived as relatively natural (non-bizarre). Judges were instructed that bizarreness was not to be equated with the ability to achieve stress on the targeted syllable and that it was possible to achieve targeted stress in a bizarre manner and possible to signal stress on the wrong word, but do so in a natural manner. Three of the four authors served as judges for the ratings of bizarreness. There was unanimous agreement as to the rank ordering of bizarreness among the speakers.

Acoustic Analysis

Fundamental Frequency. The voice fundamental frequency of the sentences produced by the dysarthric speakers was extracted from the audio recording from the neck contact microphone using a Visipitch module (Kay Elemetrics, Model 6087) and displayed on a Honeywell Visicorder (Model 1805). The audio signal was filtered prior to being analyzed by the Visipitch unit using a Crown Equalizer (Model EQ 3) to better isolate fundamental frequency and to reduce extraneous noise. This fundamental frequency analysis system was calibrated using the internal circuitry of the Visipitch unit.

The fundamental frequencies of sentences produced by the normal subjects were analyzed using a fundamental frequency software package (a clipped autocorrelation procedure developed for a DEC PDP-11/23 computer). The fundamental frequency values for five productions of stimulus sentences, *Show Sam some snow,* by five different normal speakers were also analyzed using the same procedures and equipment employed for the dysarthric speakers. The results of these analyses were compared to the computer derived values. For each word in the sentence, the peak fundamental frequency values obtained from the two fundamental frequency quantification approaches were within 5Hz.

Duration. The signal (raw waveform) from the airborne microphone was amplified and displayed via the Visicorder system. After visual inspection, the experimenter marked the initiation and termination of individual phonemes in each utterance.

Intensity. The signal from the airborne microphone was directed to the Visipitch unit without filtering. The Visipitch extracted the intensity contour which was displayed through the Visicorder system. The intensity analysis system responded linearly through the range of amplification employed in this study, thus providing accurate measures of relative syllable intensity desired for this research.

Normalized Acoustic Data

Current theory suggests (Martin, 1972) that stress patterning during normal speech production is a relational phenomenon in which the magnitude of stress applied to any given syllable can only be interpreted in comparison to the magnitude of stress applied to other syllables within the utterance. Therefore, the experimenters chose to transform all of the acoustic measures obtained for these sentences into a relational framework. This was accomplished through a normalizing procedure in which all of the absolute measures of acoustic dimensions could be viewed as percentages of the magnitude of the dimension as produced on the initial syllable of the utterance. Three strategies were employed to examine the relational patterning of selected acoustic correlates of stress. The investigators compared acoustic measures on the syllable targeted for stress with: (1) unstressed syllables within the same utterance; (2) the same syllable in the other two utterances where it was not targeted for stress; and (3) the target syllable produced by normal speakers performing the same task.

To examine the relationship between the syllable targeted for stress and other syllables within an utterance, the three acoustic parameters of interest were normalized in reference to the initial syllable of the utterance. The word *show* was selected as a referent, because this word was never targeted for primary stress. Therefore, it was assumed that the acoustic values measured in this study for *show* would be minimally affected by the stress pattern of sentences. To test this assumption, three analyses of variance were computed for the relative peak intensity, peak fundamental frequency, and duration values associated with *show* for each of the three sentences by the 20 normal speakers. Because none of the analyses yielded significant results, the assumption of similar acoustic values for *show* across stressing patterns was supported. The normalization of the fundamental frequency data is illustrated in Table 5-2. Inspection of the table reveals that in Sentence A the word *Sam* was targeted for primary stress. The peak fundamental frequency associated with *show* was assigned a score of 100%. The peak fundamental frequen-

TABLE 5-2
Normalized fundamental frequency measures (percentages) for three stressing patterns for the utterance *Show Sam some snow.*

Sentence	Targeted Stress	Show	Sam	Some	Snow
A	Sam	100	104	82	80
B	Some	100	95	103	80
C	Snow	100	95	75	94
Stress			104	103	94
Mean of Unstressed			95	78.5	80

cy scores associated with each of the other syllables in Sentence A were normalized as a percentage of the fundamental frequency value of the referent word *show*. Thus for the example, the normalized value for the fundamental frequency for the word *Sam* was 104%; for the word *some* it was 82%; and for the word *snow* it was 80%.

The second comparison of interest was the relation between a syllable targeted for primary stress and the same syllable when it was not targeted for primary stress. For example, in Sentence B, *some* was selected for primary stress, but in Sentences A and C it was not. Table 5-2 contains an example of the normalized fundamental frequency values for both stressed and unstressed syllables. Examination of the table reveals that for this normal speaker the mean normalized fundamental frequency values for unstressed productions were consistently lower than for the same syllable when it is targeted for primary stress. In this example data, the normalized peak fundamental frequency value for primary stress on *some* was 103%, while the mean value of peak fundamental frequency for *some* as an unstressed syllable was 78.5%.

Another comparison of interest was between the stressing patterns of dysarthric and normal speakers. Data from 20 normal speakers were normalized in a manner similar to that described for the dysarthric speakers. The normalized data were averaged across the normal speakers for fundamental frequency (peak and low values) and relative intensity (peak values). Thus the normalized dimensions of each dysarthric speaker could be compared to those of normal speakers.

RESULTS AND DISCUSSION

The body of the results and discussion section is comprised of a detailed description of the data from the dysarthric speakers. The utterances from the speakers serve as examples of performance strategies employed by dysarthric speakers during attempts to signal stress.

Speaker 1

Description. Speaker 1 was a 20-year-old male who had sustained a gunshot wound to the right cerebral hemisphere. He underwent a right frontal craniotomy and was comatose for 2 to 3 weeks following surgery. Residuals included left-sided hemiparesis, generalized slowness, and flattened affect. According to neurological examination, the left upper extremity was grossly ataxic and the right mildly ataxic. Neuropsychological testing indicated diffuse brain damage. This patient's dysarthric speech was judged as predominantly ataxic by the speech pathologist who described a pattern of irregular articulatory breakdowns and an overall impression of monopitch and monoloudness. Oral diadochokinetic rates were slow and marked by an irregular rhythm. When the stressing protocol was recorded, single-word intelligibility was 95%; sentence intelligibilty was 96% at a speaking rate of 82 words-per-minute (WPM) (Yorkston and Beukelman, 1981). Speaker 1 had just completed a 3-month period of speech treatment, from 18 to 21 months post onset (MPO). His chief complaint was the slowness of his speech. Attempts to increase his speaking rate resulted in unacceptable decreases in speech intelligibility. Speech treatment initially focused on achieving primary stress on targeted syllables. When given no instructions about which strategies to use, it was noted that Speaker 1 tended to exaggerate all dimensions, including sweeping changes in fundamental frequency and excessive changes in intensity. Treatment focused on achieving stress in the proper locations in sentences and minimizing the use of fundamental frequency and intensity as strategies for signaling stress. Speaker 1 was taught to rely instead on adjustments in duration. The recordings for the stressing protocol were obtained at the end of the treatment period, 21 MPO.

Perceptual Analysis. Analysis of the perceptual ratings of stress patterning indicated that judges consistently agreed that the speaker achieved primary stress on the target syllable 100% of the time. The perceptual ratings of three stress patterns for the sentence *Show Sam some snow* as produced by Speaker 1 are presented in Figure 5-2. Examination of this figure suggests that the stress patterning achieved by Speaker 1 was similar to the average pattern achieved by normal speakers. Greatest stress was perceived on the syllable targeted for primary stress in each production. Unstressed syllables (the word *some* in Sentences A and C) were distinguished from both primarily and secondarily stressed syllables.

The perceptual ratings of bizarreness indicated that the sentences produced by Speaker 1 were judged to be more bizarre than those produced

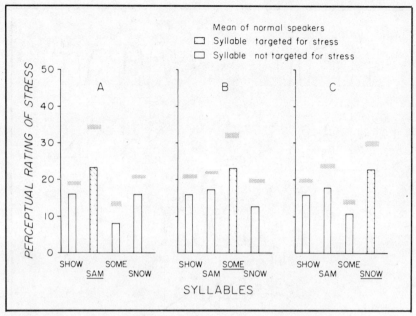

FIGURE 5-2
Mean perceptual ratings of stress across judges for normal speakers and dysarthric Speaker 1 as they produced three stressing patterns of the sentence, *Show Sam some snow.*

by the normal speaker. However, his productions were judged to be the least bizarre of the three mildly ataxic speakers represented here.

Acoustic Analysis. The relative intensity, fundamental frequency, and durational data for the sentences produced by Speaker 1 are presented in Figure 5-3A, B, and C. Examination of the figure reveals that the total sentence durations for Sentences A, B, and C are 3.7 secs., 3.4 secs., and 3.3 secs., respectively. These durations represent a speaking rate of 112 syllables per minute as compared to the normal rate on the same task of 188 syllables per minute (S.D. = 21 spm). Speaker 1 produced fundamental frequencies which ranged from 127Hz to 90Hz. Thus, he appeared to have a relatively restricted fundamental range as compared to the mean peak and low fundamental frequencies for normal speakers, also illustrated in the figure.

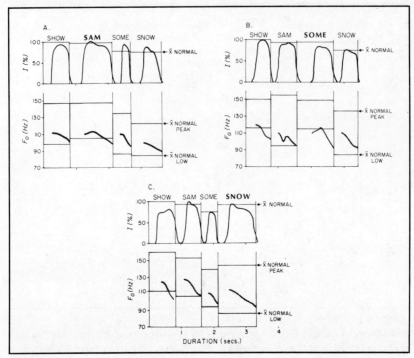

FIGURE 5-3

Shown here are the changes in relative intensity and fundamental frequency plotted against syllable duration during dysarthric Speaker 1's productions of stress patterns A, B, and C for the sentence *Show Sam some snow*. Also plotted in this figure are data showing the mean values of peak and low fundamental frequencies and peak relative intensities produced by normal speakers.

Normalized Fundamental Frequency: Normalized peak vowel fundamental frequencies for the three stressing patterns of the sentence, *Show Sam some snow* are presented in Figure 5-4A, B, and C. Also presented in this figure are the peak fundamental frequencies (ranges and means) for normal speakers, as well as the mean values of the dysarthric speaker's unstressed productions of the syllable targeted for primary stress in each utterance. Examination of this figure suggests that normal speakers typically produce a falling fundamental frequency pattern for the test sentence except for the syllable targeted for primary stress, whose fundamental frequency tends to be higher than those of adjacent syllables. Although the pattern produced by Speaker 1 is also a falling one, it appears to be flattened as compared to the pattern of normal speakers. It is possible that this relatively flat fundamental frequency pattern contributes to the perception of monotony in the productions of

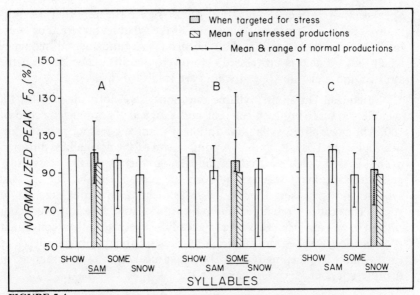

FIGURE 5-4

Peak fundamental frequency, normalized with respect to the syllable *show*, for stressing patterns A, B, and C, as Speaker 1 produced the sentence, *Show Sam some snow*. Also represented are the means and ranges of normal speakers' performance on the same task.

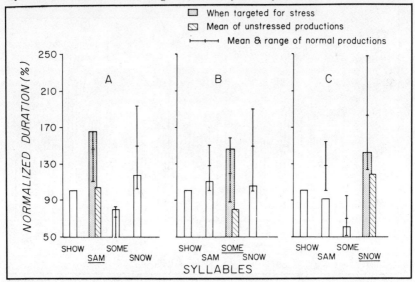

FIGURE 5-5

Syllable duration, normalized with respect to the syllable *show*, for stressing patterns A, B, and C as Speaker 1 produced the sentence *Show Sam some snow*. Also represented are the means and ranges of normal speakers' performance on the same task.

Speaker 1. A further examination of the figure suggests that the normalized peak fundamental frequencies of the syllables targeted for stress in all cases are slightly higher than the mean peak fundamental frequency when that syllable is unstressed. However, the difference between the stressed and mean unstressed values are small for Speaker 1.

Normalized Duration: Syllable durations were normalized, with the syllable *show* serving as a referent and assigned a normalized score of 100. The normalized syllable durations for three stressing patterns appear in Figure 5-5A, B, and C. A comparison of the normalized duration of the stressed syllable with the same syllable when it was unstressed suggests that Speaker 1 was exaggerating the prolongation of the stressed syllable and was using durational adjustments as a strong signaler of stress. The reader is reminded that only total syllable durations were considered in this analysis. However, typically, vowel rather than consonant prolongation was responsible for the total syllable prolongations. The final syllable lengthening typical of normal speakers is not pronounced in the utterances produced by Speaker 1.

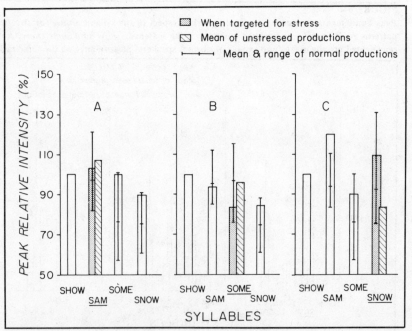

FIGURE 5-6
Peak relative intensity, normalized with respect to the syllable *show*, for stressing patterns A, B, and C, as dysarthric Speaker 1 produced the sentence, *Show Sam some snow.* Also represented are the means and ranges of normal speakers' performance on the same task.

Normalized Intensity: The peak relative intensities of each syllable were normalized relative to the word *show* which was assigned a score of 100. Figure 5-6A, B, and C illustrate this measure of relative intensity for the three stressing patterns of the sentence *Show Sam some snow.* Examination of the figure suggests that the relative intensity patterns seen in the utterances produced by dysarthric Speaker 1 were similar to the falling patterns typical of normal speakers. Only in the case of Sentence C, where stress was targeted on the final syllable, did Speaker 1 appear to use adjustments in intensity as a cue to stress.

Integration of the Acoustic Parameters: Whereas normal speakers tend to use variations in all of the parameters to signal stress in each utterance, duration was clearly the most powerful signaler of stress for dysarthric Speaker 1. His adjustments in fundamental frequency and relative intensity were minimal as compared to those used by normal speakers, except when attempting to signal stress on the final syllable. In this case, there appeared to be a trade-off between final syllable prolongation and adjustments in relative intensity. It is likely that because the final syllable is typically prolonged as compared to other syllables in the utterance, durational adjustments are not as powerful in signaling stress as they are in nonfinal sentence positions (Klatt, 1975; Oller, 1973). If this is the case, then another strategy for signaling stress must be employed. Speaker 1 used an increase in relative intensity.

Implications for Speaker 1. The data presented here are taken from samples produced by Speaker 1 at the end of a period of treatment that focused on achieving accurate stressing patterns. Pretreatment acoustic measures were unavailable. Speaker 1 was consistently able to signal stress on the targeted syllable. He did so using the strategies he was taught. For this speaker treatment was terminated because he became active in a prevocational program in another city. If he had continued treatment, the next phase would have focused on attempts to reduce bizarreness. The investigators judged that bizarreness in the speech of Speaker 1 was the result of two factors. The first was his slowed speaking rate. Previous attempts to increase speaking rate in Speaker 1 were unsuccessful, as the efforts resulted in undesirable decreases in intelligibility. The second factor contributing to bizarreness was the habitually flat fundamental frequency contour. This factor may have been more amenable to treatment than speaking rate. If treatment had continued, slight, unexaggerated changes in fundamental frequency would have been re-introduced and the effect of these modifications on bizarreness assessed.

Speaker 2

Description. Speaker 2 was a.29-year-old male who experienced an episode of septic shock with secondary renal failure that left him with residual dysarthria, mild upper extremity weakness, and an ataxic gait pattern. His speech pattern was described by his speech-language pathologist as predominately ataxic. All speech sounds could be produced correctly in isolation. Connected speech was marked by rapid rate, failure to achieve articulatory targets, and harsh voice quality. Oral diadochokinetic movements were slow and dysrhythmic. Speech treatment was initiated 2-months post onset. At the time, sentence intelligibility was 26% and single word intelligibility was 56% (Yorkston and Beukelman, 1981). Speaker 2 completed a 2-month period of daily speech treatment with an initial focus on separation of words, inclusion of final consonants, and reduction in bursts of excessive loudness. At the time of recording, 4 MPO, his sentence intelligibility was 98% at 78 WPM. He received no specific training in producing normal stressing prior to his departure from the rehabilitation center.

Perceptual Analysis. Analysis of the perceptual ratings of stress indicated that Speaker 2 successfully achieved stress on the targeted

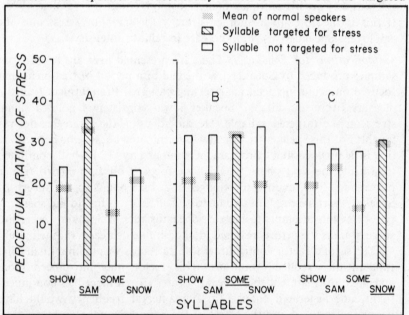

FIGURE 5-7
Mean perceptual ratings of stress across judges for normal speakers and dysarthric Speaker 2, as they produced three stressing patterns of the sentence, *Show Sam some snow.*

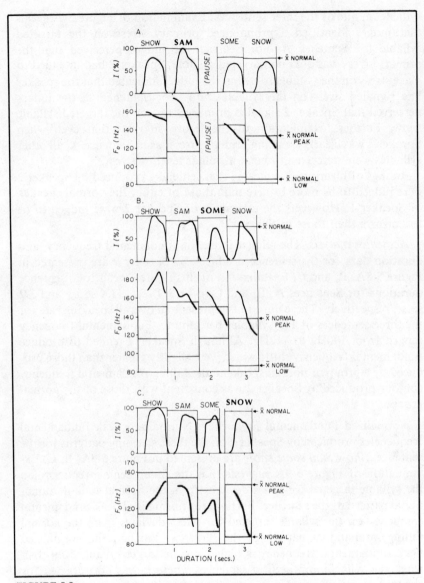

FIGURE 5-8

Shown are the changes in relative intensity and fundamental frequency plotted against syllable duration during dysarthric Speaker 2's productions of stress patterns A, B, and C for the sentence *Show Sam some snow*. Also plotted in this figure are data showing the mean values of peak and low fundamental frequencies and peak relative intensities produced by normal speakers.

syllable on one of the three sentences. Examination of Figure 5-7 reveals that judges identified a pronounced primary stress on the targeted syllable for Sentence A. For Sentence B, judges perceived that the primary stress was on a nontargeted syllable. Speaker 2 had intended to place stress on the syllable *some* but the judges indicated that the speaker had signaled stress on the syllable *snow*. For Sentence C, the judges perceived that Speaker 2 signaled primary stress on the targeted syllable *snow*. Further, examination of the figure suggests that even when Speaker 2 was clearly signaling primary stress, as in Sentence A, all other syllables were perceived to be at a similar level of stress.

Ratings of bizarreness indicated that sentences produced by Speaker 2 were judged to be more bizarre than those of either the normal speaker or Speaker 1. However, the utterances of Speaker 2 were judged to be less bizarre than those of Speaker 3.

Acoustic Analysis. The relative intensity, fundamental frequency, and duration data for the sentence produced by Speaker 2 are presented in Figure 5-8A, B, and C. Examination of this figure reveals total sentence durations for Sentences A, B, and C to be 3.9 secs., 3.4 secs., and 3.2 secs., respectively. These durations represent an overall speaking rate for the three sentences of 115 syllables per minute. Fundamental frequency ranged from 190Hz to 112Hz. Although Speaker 2 tended to produce fundamental frequency shifts which were slightly greater than those produced by a group of normal speakers, the falling fundamental frequency contour produced by Speaker 2 was consistent with those of the normal group.

Normalized Fundamental Frequency: Normalized peak fundamental frequencies produced by Speaker 2 on the three stressing patterns for the sentence, *Show Sam some snow* are presented in Figure 5-9A, B, C. Examination of Figure 5-9A suggests that the fundamental frequency on the syllable targeted for stress deviates from the normal falling intonational pattern of the sentence. Further, the normalized peak fundamental frequency on the syllable targeted for stress deviates from the normal falling intonational pattern of the sentence. Further, the normalized peak fundamental frequency is higher on the target syllable *Sam* than when the syllable appeared in sentences where it was not targeted for primary stress. Therefore, fundamental frequency shifts appeared to signal stress in the only sentence in which judges clearly perceived that increased stress was produced in the targeted location. Neither in Sentence B nor C, did fundamental frequency serve as a cue to the location of the stressed syllable.

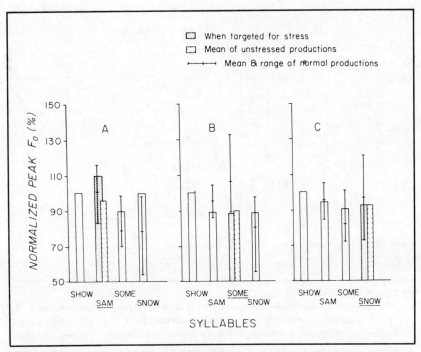

FIGURE 5-9
Peak fundamental frequency, normalized with respect to the syllable *show*, for stressing patterns A, B, and C as dysarthric Speaker 2 produced the sentence *Show Sam some snow*. Also represented are the means and ranges of normal speakers' performance on the same task.

Normalized Duration: Normalized syllable durations for Sentences A, B, and C appear in Figure 5-10A, B, and C. Examination of this figure suggests a nearly equal syllable duration regardless of intended stress or syllable position. In other words, syllables that are targeted for primary stress are neither longer nor shorter than their unstressed counterparts and sentence-final syllables. The only durational adjustments that Speaker 2 made were insertions for interword pauses immediately following the syllable targeted for stress in Sentence A and just prior to the syllable targeted for stress in Sentence C.

Normalized Intensity: The normalized, peak relative intensities of each syllable are illustrated in Figure 5-11A, B, C. Examination of the figure suggests that Speaker 2 produced an exaggerated increase in relative intensity to signal the stress location in Sentence A. In Sentence B, a lack of deviation from the normal falling contour pattern may have contributed to the failure to signal stress on the targeted syllable *some*. Instead,

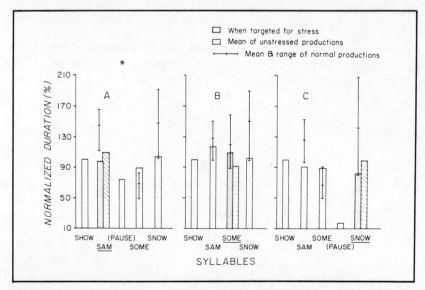

FIGURE 5-10
Syllable duration, normalized with respect to the syllable *show* for stressing patterns A, B, and C as dysarthric Speaker 2 produced the sentence *Show Sam some snow*. Also represented are the means and ranges of normal speakers' performance on the same task.

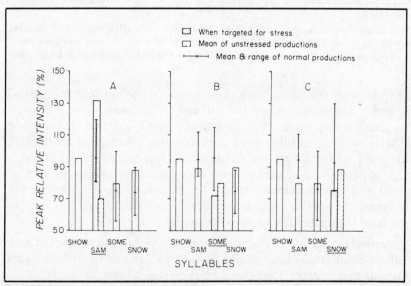

FIGURE 5-11
Peak relative intensity, normalized with respect to the syllable *show* for stressing patterns A, B, and C, as dysarthric Speaker 2 produced the sentence *Show Sam some snow*. Also represented are the means and ranges of normal speakers' performance on the same task.

judges may have been misled by the increase in relative intensity of the final syllable, leading them to identify primary stress on the syllable *snow*. In Sentence C, relative intensity of the syllable targeted for stress does not differ from the falling intensity pattern which is characteristic of an unstressed production.

Integration of the Acoustic Parameters: Each of the three stressing patterns for the sentence *Show Sam some snow* produced by Speaker 2 is perceptually unique. Therefore, the strategies which contribute to each perceptual pattern will be discussed separately. In Sentence A, a pronounced primary stress is perceived on the target syllable. Speaker 2 appears to control three acoustic features in order to produce this perceptual result. The first adjustment is an exaggerated shift in relative intensity on the syllable targeted for stress; the second is the insertion of an interword pause following the syllable targeted for stress; and the third is a moderate increase in peak fundamental frequency on the syllable targeted for stress. In Sentence B, judges perceived a flattened stressing pattern, but in this case, slight increases in stressing were noted on the syllable which had been targeted for stress. Because syllable stress location was not signaled with either intensity or durational adjustments, the increase in fundamental frequency of the final syllable apparently was responsible for perception of a slight increase in stress in the final syllable.

Implications for Speaker 2. A number of implications for treatment can be drawn from the data presented here. With Speaker 2, the first phase of treatment would focus on training him to consistently signal stress on the targeted syllable. While exploring reliable strategies that this patient could use to signal stress, care should also be taken to train strategies which would not increase the bizarreness of the utterances. Training Speaker 2 to make durational adjustments from syllable-to-syllable might be a productive avenue for exploration. Speaker 2's pattern of nearly equal duration for all syllables probably contributes in an important way to the judges' rating that the amount of stress on syllables produced by this speaker was "excess and equal." The durational pattern may have contributed to the judges rating this speaker as more bizarre than Speaker 1. The only durational adjustments that Speaker 2 made were to insert interword pauses preceding or following the syllable targeted for stress. A more natural durational adjustment would have included prolongation of the stressed vowel and a reduction of the duration of the unstressed vowels. Reduction in vowel duration may not be an option for some ataxic dysarthric speakers because of their coordination deficits. In these cases, a vowel modification in the form of vowel reduction (schwa substitution) and not an adjustment in duration may be useful in "unstressing" a syllable. Data from this study revealed that normal speakers often omitted the vowel in the unstressed production of the word *some*. The dysarthric speakers never used vowel-omission-syllable reduction as a stressing strategy. Training Speaker 2 to make durational adjustments might go hand-in-hand with training him to minimize the use of stressing features he has difficulty controlling, specifically intensity. Speaker 2 relied heavily on intensity adjustments to signal stress, a strategy that does not appear to be important for normal speakers. Normal speakers rarely use intensity alone to signal stress. When intensity is used to signal stress it is used in conjunction with adjustments in fundamental frequency and duration. Specifically, Speaker 2 might be trained first to increase the duration of words he wishes to stress. Once this is accomplished, he might be trained also to reduce selected unstressed syllables, by syllable reduction-vowel omission.

Speaker 3

Description. Speaker 3 was a 24-year-old male who sustained a severe brain injury approximately 9 years prior to participation in this research project. Initially, he was described as aphonic, but during recovery he began to use speech as his primary means of communication. At 1-year post injury, his speech was characterized as predominantly ataxic with reduced intelligibility, poor respiratory support for speech, discoordination of respiration and phonation, and monotonous pitch. During the period from 1- to 9-years post onset, detailed information was not available. However, it appeared that speech continued to improve. At the time of recording, both single-word and sentence intelligibility were 98% (Yorkston and Beukelman, 1981). Although prosodic patterns were described as bizarre, Speaker 3 was able to adjust fundamental frequency and intensity to signal stress. He had not been actively involved in a speech training program for a number of years prior to recording.

Perceptual Analysis. Analysis of the perceptual ratings of stress indicated that Speaker 3 successfully signaled syllable stress location on the targeted syllables of each of the three sentences. Examination of Figure 5-12 reveals that judges identified a pronounced primary stress on the targeted syllable for all sentences. This primary stressing pattern was set against the relatively flattened pattern of unstressed syllables. There was little distinction between syllables which normally receive secondary stress and those which are normally unstressed.

After listening to the three sentences produced by Speaker 3 for this project, his speech was judged to be the most bizarre of the three speakers. In fact, bizarreness was one of the most predominant characteristics of his speech pattern.

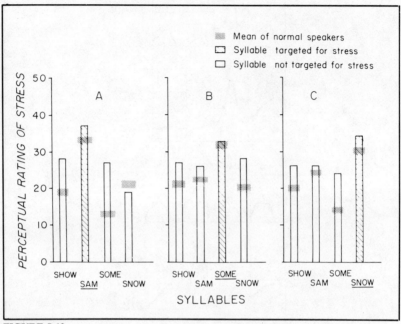

FIGURE 5-12
Mean perceptual ratings of stress across judges for normal speakers and dysarthric Speaker 3, as they produce three stressing patterns of the sentence, *Show Sam some snow*.

Acoustic Analysis. The relative intensity, fundamental frequency and durational data for the sentences produced by Speaker 3 are presented in Figure 5-13A, B, and C. Examination of this figure reveals that the total durations for Sentences A, B, and C were 3.7 secs., 3.9 secs., and 3.2 secs., respectively. These durations represent an average speaking rate of 112 syllables per minute. Fundamental frequency ranged from 155 to 85Hz. At times, the fundamental frequency shifts for a single syllable extended over nearly the entire range. For example, when the syllable *some* was targeted for stress in Sentence B, the fundamental frequency contour followed a rise-fall pattern from 110 to 144 to 90Hz. In terms of intensity, the syllables targeted for stress were much more intense than the other syllables.

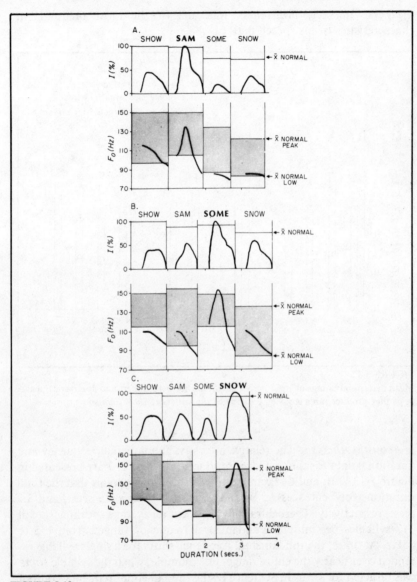

FIGURE 5-13
Shown here are the changes in relative intensity and fundamental frequency plotted against syllable duration during dysarthric Speaker 3's productions of stress patterns A, B, and C for the sentence *Show Sam some snow*. Also plotted in this figure are data showing the mean values of peak and low fundamental frequencies and peak relative intensities produced by normal speakers.

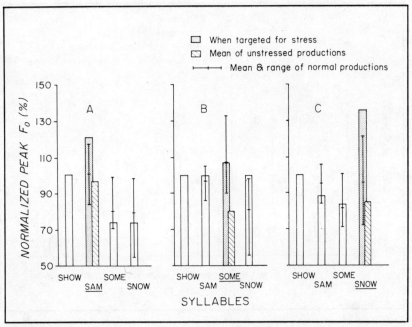

FIGURE 5-14
Peak fundamental frequency, normalized with respect to the syllable *show*, for stressing patterns A, B, and C, as dysarthric Speaker 3 produced the sentence *Show Sam some snow.* Also represented are the means and ranges of normal speakers' performance on the same task.

Normalized Fundamental Frequency: The normalized peak vowel fundamental frequencies produced by Speaker 3 on the three token sentences, are presented in Figure 5-14A, B, and C. Examination of this figure suggests that in all cases, the normalized fundamental frequency values on the syllable targeted for stress deviated from the expected falling fundamental frequency pattern for these sentences. Further, these fundamental frequency shifts were exaggerated, falling outside the normal range for Sentences A and C.

Normalized Duration: Normalized syllable durations for the Sentences A, B, and C appear in Figure 5-15A, B, and C. Examination of these figures shows nearly equal syllable duration regardless of intended stress or syllable position. With the possible exception of Sentence B, Speaker 3 did not appear to be using durational adjustments to signal stress. Unlike normal speakers, he did not tend to prolong the final syllable of the utterance relative to other syllables within the utterance.

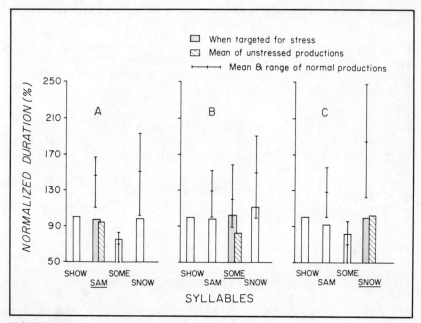

FIGURE 5-15
Syllable duration, normalized with respect to the syllable *show* for stressing patterns A, B, and C as dysarthric Speaker 3 produced the sentence *Show Sam some snow.* Also represented are the means and ranges of normal speakers' performance on the same task.

Normalized Intensity: Normalized, peak relative intensities for the syllables in each sentence are illustrated in Figure 5-16A, B, and C. Examination of this figure suggests that Speaker 3 produced exaggerated relative intensity increases to signal stress in all sentences. In all cases, the intensity of the syllable targeted for stress was well outside the normal range. For example in Sentence A, the normalized intensity for the stressed syllable *Sam* was 233% of the referent syllable *show*, yet the following syllable *some* was only 44% of the intensity of the referent syllable. Thus, one of the two adjacent syllables greatly exceeded the normal range while the other fell well below it. These large shifts in relative intensity no doubt contributed to the perceived bizarreness of the utterances produced by Speaker 3.

Integration of the Acoustic Parameters: Results of the perceptual analysis revealed that Speaker 3 achieved a stressing pattern that was characterized by a pronounced and unequivocal signaling of primary stress for all sentences. Acoustically, this pattern was signaled by consistent and exaggerated shifts in peak fundmental frequency and relative intensity. The relatively equal syllable durations within these utterances

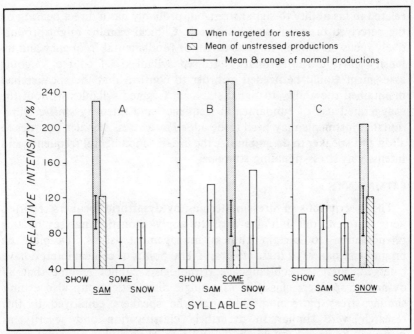

FIGURE 5-16

Peak relative intensity, normalized with respect to the syllable *show* **for stressing patterns A, B, and C, as dysarthric Speaker 3 produced the sentence,** *Show Sam some snow.* **Also represented are the means and ranges of normal speakers' performance on the same task.**

suggests that Speaker 3 was not making use of durational adjustments to signal stress. Perhaps judges were able to identify targeted stress so clearly because this speaker employed exaggerated stress signaling strategies. Of equal importance, he did not mislead the judges by placing stress on nontargeted syllables.

Implications for Speaker 3. A number of clinical decisions can be made on the basis of the perceptual and acoustic data previously presented. Treatment focusing on decreasing the bizarreness of Speaker 3's stress patterning may be a useful approach. The relatively high rating of bizarreness for this speaker may have been the result of a number of acoustic features; specifically the exaggerated use of fundamental frequency and intensity as signalers of stress may have contributed to the overall bizarreness of the speaker's speech pattern.

In addition, this speaker not only failed to prolong the syllables targeted for stress, but also failed to shorten typically unstressed words such as *some* or to prolong utterance-final syllables. The failure of this speaker to make a number of durational adjustments may not be directly related to his ability to signal stress but probably has a direct bearing on the perceived bizarreness of his speech. Clinical training might productively focus on diminishing the extent of fundamental frequency and intensity shifts during primarily stressed syllables. Of course, ongoing assessment would be needed in order to confirm that the speaker had maintained the ability to signal stress on targeted syllables without the exaggerated use of fundamental frequency and intensity shifts. Durational adjustments may need to be added as a stress signaler in order to allow this speaker to de-emphasize the use of fundamental frequency and intensity as stress-signaling strategies.

COMMENTS

The descriptions of stress patterning by dysarthric speakers reported here represent our initial efforts to apply acoustic analyses of this phenomenon to certain clinical management issues. Despite the preliminary nature of these efforts, several points of clinical interest have emerged. First, speech-language pathologists cannot assume that all dysarthric speakers classified in a single diagnostic group also exhibit similar stress patterning. Although the speakers employed in this research were similar in dysarthria classification and severity as measured by speech intelligibility and rate, their ability to signal stress accurately on targeted syllables and the strategies they used for signaling stress differed. Therefore, use of a standard treatment approach based on type of dysarthria alone does not appear to be appropriate. Instead, the differences between the speakers led us to recommend unique treatment approaches for each.

Second, the speech-language pathologist's assessment of the adequacy of stress patterning must consider more than accuracy alone. Although accuracy reflects how successful the speaker was in achieving stress on the targeted syllable and is a necessary indicator of severity of the prosodic disruption, it must be viewed in relation to the bizarreness of the utterance. Consideration of bizarreness is especially critical in treatment planning because some strategies used by a particular dysarthric speaker to signal stress may be judged as more bizarre than others.

One important purpose of any assessment tool is to give guidelines for the sequencing of treatment. Figure 5-17 illustrates some of the questions that might be answered by perceptual and acoustic analysis of performance on a stress patterning task. Perhaps the most fundamental question is, "Does the speaker know where the locus of stress should be?" If the answer to this question is "no," then training in the recognition of prominence is appropriate. If the answer is "yes," then a second question would be asked. Does the speaker achieve primary stress on the

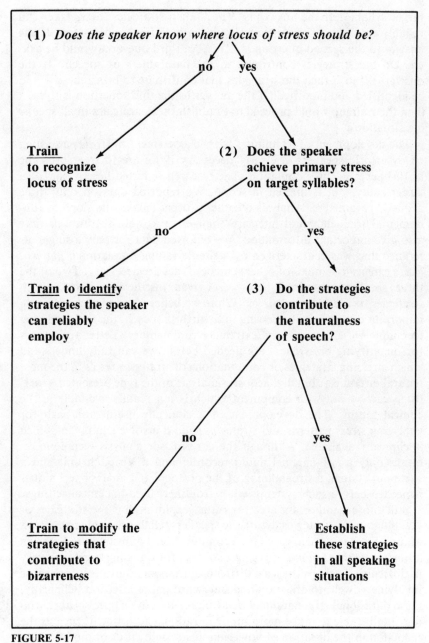

FIGURE 5-17
Sequence of assessment questions and training tasks for stress patterning in dysarthric speakers.

target syllable? If the answer is "no," then strategies the speaker can reliably employ to signal stress should be identified and trained. If the answer to the second question is "yes," a third question would be asked. Do the strategies contribute to the naturalness of speech? If the answer is "no," then the strategies that contribute to bizarreness would be identified and modified. If the answer to the third question is "yes," then the training would proceed to establish these strategies in all speaking situations.

The development of techniques for the assessment of stress patterning of dysarthric speakers is clearly necessary if we are to treat prosodic disturbances in this population. The research reported here is part of a larger study, but is limited in scope. We reported data on only three acoustic parameters. Analysis of other aspects such as the slope of fundamental frequency and intensity changes or vowel substitutions may also give important information. We reported data for only a single utterance that was characterized by a simple falling intonational pattern. More extensive samples of other sentence types are necessary. Two of the three speakers examined here were given instructions about which strategies to use to signal stress. While we believe that bizarreness is an important dimension of stressing in dysarthric speech, the rank ordering technique we employed was extremely rudimentary. Better techniques for quantifying bizarreness are needed before we can fully understand which stressing strategies or combinations of strategies result in the most natural utterances. Finally, acoustic analysis of the type presented here is often carried out with equipment which is not readily available in the clinical setting. The development of a clinically useful approach for analyzing stress patterns and strategies should involve equipment which is clinically available. Although the core of our analysis technique requires only a two-channel audio recorder and a Visipitch unit and a write-out system, a streamlining of the protocol and analysis techniques is needed before such systems will be routinely used in clinical settings.

Still another important area for future exploration is the strategies or combination of strategies dysarthric speakers reliably are able to control. Many of our treatment tasks focus on durational adjustments. Yet even adjustments that fall into this single strategy for signaling stress may vary in difficulty. Perhaps the least difficult durational adjustments are those involving vowel prolongation and interword pause insertion. Clinically, these durational strategies may be available to a dysarthric speaker who may not be able to make more subtle durational adjustments such as the reduction in the duration of vowels in unstressed words or modification in consonant duration.

There appears to be an increasing professional interest in the clinical assessment and treatment of the prosodic anomalies which interfere with the communication effectiveness of dysarthric speakers. The clinical tools and approaches to be used in this effort are few and largely untested. Expertise in the areas of acoustics, physiology, motor training, and communication effectiveness appear necessary to move this effort forward. Progress in this area requires the cooperation of basic speech scientists and clinical speech pathologists, for neither group alone appears to have the necessary knowledge and resources.

REFERENCES

Atkinson, J. E. Inter- and intraspeaker variability in fundamental voice frequency. *Journal of the Acoustical Society of America,* 1976, *60,* (2), 440-445.

Barnes, G. J. Suprasegmental and prosodic considerations in motor speech disorders. In W. Berry (Ed.), *Clinical dysarthria.* San Diego: College-Hill Press, 1983, 57-68.

Bleakley, D. The effect of fundamental frequency variation on the perception of stress in German. *Phonatica,* 1973, *28,* 42-59.

Caligiuri, M. P., & Murry, T. The use of visual feedback to enhance prosodic control in dysarthria. In W. Berry (Ed.), *Clinical dysarthria.* San Diego: College-Hill Press, 1983, 267-282.

Chomsky, N., & Halle, M. *The sound pattern of English.* New York: Harper & Row, 1968.

Chueng, J. Y., Holden, A. D., & Minifie, F. D. Computer estimation and modeling of linguistic stress patterns in speech (Tech. Rep. 108). Seattle: Department of Electrical Engineering, University of Washington, 1973, 150.

Darley, F. L., Aronson, A. E., & Brown, J. K. Clusters of deviant speech dimensions in the dysarthrias. *Journal of Speech and Hearing Research,* 1969, *12,* 462-469. (a)

Darley, F. L., Aronson, A. E., & Brown, J. R. Differential diagnostic patterns of dysarthria. *Journal of Speech and Hearing Research,* 1969, *12,* 246-269. (b)

Darley, F. L., Aronson, A. E., & Brown, J. R. *Motor speech disorders,* Philadelphia: Saunders, 1975.

Fry, D. B. Duration and intensity as physical correlates of linguistic stress. *The Journal of the Acoustical Society of America,* 1955, *27,* (4), 765-768.

Kent, R. D., & Rosenbek, J. C. Prosodic disturbance and neurologic lesion. *Brain and Language,* 1982, *15,* 259-291.

Klatt, D. H. Vowel lengthening is syntactically determined in a connected discourse. *Journal of Phonetics,* 1975, 129-140.

Lea, W. A., Medress, M. F., & Skinner, T. E. *Prosodic aids to speech recognition I: Basic algorithms and stress studies.* (Univac Rep. PX7940) St. Paul, MN: Univac Park, 1972.

Lehiste, I. *Suprasegmentals,* Cambridge: MIT Press, 1970.

Lieberman, P. Some acoustic correlates of word stress in American English. *Journal of the Acoustical Society of America.* 1960, *32,* 451-454.

Martin, J.G. Rhythmic (hierarchical) versus serial structure in speech and other behavior. *Psychology Review,* 1972, *79,* 487-509.

Morton, J., & Jassem, W. Acoustic correlates of stress. *Language and Speech,* 1965, *8,* 159-181.

Murry, T. The production of stress in three types of dysarthric speech. In W. Berry (Ed.), *Clinical dysarthria.* College-Hill Press, 1983, 69-84.

Netsell, R. Speech physiology. In F. D. Minifie, T. J. Hixon, & F. Williams (Eds.), *Normal aspects of speech, hearing and language.* Englewood Cliffs, NJ: Prentice-Hall, 1973.

Ohman, S. Word and sentence intonation. A quantitative model. *Speech Transmission Laboratory QPSR,* 2-3 Stockholm: Royal Institute of Technology, 1967, 20-54.

Oller, D. K. The effects of position in utterance on speech segment duration in English. *Journal of the Acoustical Society of America,* 1973, *54,* 1235-1247.

O'Shaughnessy, D. Linguistic features in fundamental frequency patterns. *Journal of Phonetics,* 1979, *7,* 119-145.

Rosenbek, J. C., & LaPointe, L. L. The dysarthrias: Description, diagnosis, and treatment. In D. F. Johns, (Ed.), *Clinical management of neurogenic communicative disorders.* Boston: Little, Brown & Company, 1978, 251-310.

Simmons, N. N. Acoustic analysis of ataxic dysarthria. An approach to monitoring treatment. In W. Berry, (Ed.), *Clinical dysarthria.* San Diego: College-Hill Press, 1983, 183-295.

Yorkston, K. M., & Beukelman, D. R. *Assessment of intelligibility of dysarthric speech.* Tigard, OR: C.C. Publications, 1981.

ACKNOWLEDGMENTS

This study was supported in part by National Institute of Handicapped Research Grant #G008200020, Department of Education. The authors wish to thank Chris Prall, Ann Borst, and Tamara Hoover for their assistance.

6

Relationships between Perceptual Ratings and Acoustic Measures of Hypokinetic Speech

Christy L. Ludlow
Celia J. Bassich

INTRODUCTION

Neurologists diagnose neuromotor disorders on the basis of medical history and the pattern of signs and symptoms of neurological impairment. Sensory, motor, and cranial nerve functioning are assessed by clinical examination. Complicating pathologies are ruled out through laboratory tests that assess such things as cerebrospinal fluid or with imaging techniques such as CT scan results. The presence or absence of certain pathophysiological states or movement disorders such as bradykinesia, rigidity, flaccidity, dyskinesia, ataxia, hyperreflexia, chorea, and tremor at rest and during movement are important in the diagnosis. Speech symptoms, therefore, are one aspect of the patient's motor functioning and are reflective of the neurological disorder, as are other motor functions such as walking and writing. Patients with Parkinson's disease, a hypokinetic movement disorder, have similar movement initiation problems, with acceleration of rate and poverty of range of movement in speaking, writing, and walking. By contrast, in dyskinesia, a hyperkinetic movement disorder, involuntary movements of the limbs, neck, and trunk disturb the rhythm and rate of motor activities including speech.

As neurologists use an inventory of signs and symptoms for identification of neuromotor disorders, so Darley, Aronson, and Brown (1969) were able to develop a perceptual rating scale on 38 dimensions which could differentiate between the patterns of speech symptoms associated with different types of neurological disease. The neurological examination and the perceptual speech rating system of Darley et al. (1969) share limitations, however, when used for clinical research. Both are qualitative and depend on the clinical perception and experience of the examiner. They are not quantitative and have limited measurement resolution for reflecting different degrees of impairment in motor or speech functioning necessary for the assessment of treatment effects (Henderson, Sandowsky, Shapiro, & Van Buren, 1973).

When embarking on a program of clinical research aimed at determining the efficacy of pharmacological agents for improving speech production in neurological disease, we required an objective and quantitative method for evaluating the degree and pattern of speech impairment. Since the perceptual system of Darley et al. (1969) identified speech attributes valid for differentiating between different types of dysarthria, we decided to build on that base by using speech tasks that would isolate the same speech attributes. Canter's studies (1963, 1965a, 1965b) of the speech and respiratory functioning of patients with Parkinson's disease demonstrated how these patients differed from normal on several nonspeech tasks assessing the motor support for speech. Lehiste's (1965) extensive acoustic study of dysarthric patients' speech productions demonstrated that acoustic analysis could be a useful tool for measuring speech impairment.

Using this research as a base we embarked on the development of a system for measuring of speech impairment in neurologic disease which would accomplish the following:

(1.) Differentiate between normal and dysarthric speakers;

(2.) Differentiate between the patterns of speech impairment associated with different types of neuromotor disorders; and

(3.) Be sensitive to different degrees of impairment and the effects of treatment for dysarthria.

To accomplish these objectives we developed speech tasks aimed at assessing both the maximum rate and range of movement of the speech articulators as well as the use of the same articulatory movements for linguistic expression. Procedures for acoustic analysis were developed to provide objective and quantitative measures of degree of impairment. A previous study compared patients with normal controls and different groups of patients, to identify valid measures for the differentiation of types of speech production impairments associated with different neurological disorders (Ludlow & Bassich, 1983).

In this study, the relevance of this acoustic measurement system to those aspects of speech production found by Darley et al. (1969) to be clinically significant was to be determined in patients with Parkinson's disease. The validity of the acoustic system would be demonstrated if perceptual ratings similar to those of Darley et al. (1969) were related to acoustic measures of speech performance in the same patients.

Subjects

Twelve patients with idiopathic Parkinson's disease were examined by a neurologist prior to speech testing and determined to be clearly hypokinetic with tremor, rigidity, and no dyskinesia. All were ambulatory, had bilateral movement problems, and complained of speech difficulties. All were receiving medication at the time of testing in relatively low dosages of levodopa, carbidopa, and/or bromocriptine. Normal controls with no history of neurologic, otolaryngologic, or speech and language disorders were selected and matched for sex and age (within 6 years). Each group consisted of eight male and four female subjects. The mean age for the patient group was 59.68 and 59.85 years for the controls, with a range in age from 44 to 76 years.

Speech Recordings

Subjects were recorded in a sound treated environment with a head-held Electret condenser microphone at a constant mouth-to-microphone distance of 7 inches. Prior to speech testing, a 1000Hz calibration tone was read at the face of the subject's microphone with a General Radio Sound Level Meter. A 13-minute instruction tape provided the speech items for imitation, which included: extended phonation of the vowels /ɑ/ and /i/; imitation of two sentences (A) *When he comes home, we'll feed him.* and (B) *Did he go to the right, or to the left?* at regular and fast speech rates; rapid repetition for 7 seconds of the vowels /ɑ/,/i/,/i-u/, /u-ɑ/ and the syllables /pɑ/,/tɑ/,/kɑ/,/pɑ-tɑ/ and /pɑ-kɑ/; production of a vowel or syllable rapidly as possible after a click; imitation of a low to high pitch glide on the vowel /ɑ/; imitation of pitch contour in a sentence; imitation of four loudness levels: soft, normal, loud and shout of the vowel /ɑ/ and the word *no*; and imitating the following sentences with word boundary contrasts.

(C₁) *It was a blue bell.*
(C₂) *It was a bluebell.*
(D₁) *They will sail boats.*

(D₂) *They were sailboats.*
(E₁) *She said a cross word.*
(E₂) *She did a crossword.*

Both the instructions, the calibration tone, and each subject's responses were recorded via a Nagra IV-S tape recorder on Scotch low-noise tape.

Perceptual assessments. Nineteen speech attributes reported by Darley et al. (1969) to be impaired in various types of dysarthria associated with basal ganglia disease were selected for study: overall rate, increasing rate, short rushes, inappropriate silences, variable rate, hypernasality, wet hoarseness, strain strangled voice, breathy voice, harsh voice, reduced stress, excess stress, pitch level, pitch breaks (i.e. uncontrolled pitch variation), monopitch, overall loudness, uncontrolled loudness variation, monoloudness, and imprecise consonants. An additional parameter frequently noted in neuropathogies of speech, "glottal fry," was added. Ten of the parameters were those noted by Darley et al. (1969) to be most deviant in the speech of patients with parkinsonism: monopitch, reduced stress, monoloudness, imprecise consonants, inappropriate silences, short rushes, harsh voice quality, breathy voice (continuous), pitch level, and variable rate.

Definitions for the 20 perceptual rating categories used in this study are in Appendix 6-A. Seventeen attributes were rated between 1 and 7 with 1 representing no abnormality, 2 representing mild and inconsistent (occurring less than 75% of the time), 3 representing moderate and inconsistent, 4 representing mild and consistent (occurring more than 75% of the time), 5 representing moderate and consistent, 6 representing severe and consistent, and 7 representing complete dysfunction. Pitch level, loudness level, and overall rate were judged on 13-point scales with 7 being normal, 1 being the lowest extreme of too low, too soft or too slow respectively, and 13 being the highest extreme of too high, too loud, or too fast. To provide a common reference for judging pitch and loudness, synthesized /ɑ/ vowels were recorded with fundamental frequencies of 100Hz for males and 200Hz for females and played to listeners at 80dB SPL re .0002 dynes/cm² prior to listening to each subject tape.

Three speech pathology graduate students participated as listeners. Prior to the study, they were given 20, 1-hour sessions of listening to training tapes of dysarthric and normal speakers and were required to reach an inter-rater, intra-class correlation coefficient of .85 or greater on each of the 20 rating categories.

Following training, the three raters listened to the 24 experimental tapes of the control and Parkinson patients played in random order without any identification regarding pathology or normalcy. Listeners were 2 feet from a tape recorder in a sound-controlled room, with the playback level of the calibration tone set at the same sound pressure level at the listener's ears as was measured at the subject's microphone during speech recording. The mean rating for each subject for each attribute was computed for analysis.

Acoustic assessment. The following acoustic analyses and measurement techniques were used for each speech recording without knowledge of speaker's identity.

(1) Extended phonation length in seconds was measured five times with a stop watch and the modal value determined for the vowels /ɑ/ and /i/.

(2) The peak intensity level in decibels re .0002 dynes/cm² sound pressure level was measured from graphic level recordings of the four loudness level productions (soft, regular, loud, and shout) for the vowel /ɑ/ and the word *no*. The sound level meter intensity reading of the calibration tone provided the reference in decibels for determining the intensity level of a subject's productions. The range in decibels between soft and loud and between soft and shout were computed.

(3) To measure average intensity in sentences, the peak intensity level in decibels of the final word in four sentences were averaged. (A) *When he comes home we'll feed him* (regular rate), (B) *Did he go to the right or to the left* (regular rate), (C₁) *It was a blue bell* and (E₁) *She said a cross word*.

(4) The latency of speech initiation following a click was measured with an x-y digitizer from sound spectrograms. The distance from initiation of the click to initiation of phonation was measured in centimeters and converted to seconds.

(5) The total times for the production of sentences (A) and (B) at regular and fast rates, were measured from wide-band spectrograms. The time from speech initiation to termination was measured in cms and converted to seconds with an x-y digitizer for the regular rate and fast rate productions of each sentence. The difference in total time for the two productions of each sentence were also computed.

(6) From sound spectrograms of vowel and syllable repetitions, the following measures were made: the number of vowel or syllable productions in 5 sec; the number of gaps in phonation (on-off phonations) in 5 sec; the number of productions of a vowel or syllable in the first 1.5 sec of repetition; the number of productions of a vowel or syllable in the last 1.5 sec of repetition (4 to 5.5 sec after starting repetition); and, the number of repetitions in the last

1.5 sec minus the number in the first 1.5 sec (as a measure of change in rate).

(7) Duration changes in syllable lengths and interword pauses, to distinguish word barriers, were measured from sound spectrograms. Three pairs of sentences (C_1 and C_2, D_1 and D_2, and E_1 and E_2) contained the same words either as two separate words or as a compound noun. The distance from initiation of the first word to initiation of the second was measured with an x-y digitizer in cm and converted to seconds for each of the six sentences. The difference in time between the interword intervals in the two-word (equal stress) and compound noun (unequal stress) conditions was computed to determine the duration changes made by the subjects to mark word barriers.

(8) Spectrogams made using a scale magnifier to expand the region between 0 and 550Hz were used to measure fundamental frequency (f_o). Fifty and 500-Hz tones were used to calibrate the x-y digitizer in hertz. The f_o value was measured at designated points along the f_o contour with the x-y digitizer.

(9) To measure mean f_o in sentences, the peak f_o values on the six nouns in the sentences C_1, D_1, and E_1 were averaged.

(10) Change in f_o with stress contrasts, between the two word and compound noun conditions was measured by the following procedures. The peak f_o values of the two words in sentences C_1, D_1, and E_1 were measured and the difference in f_o values between the two nouns within each sentence was computed.

Similarly, the difference in peak f_o between the first syllable and the second syllable in the compound noun condition in sentences C_2, D_2, and E_2 was measured and the differences between the f_o values of the first and second syllables were computed. F_o changes with stress changes were measured by computing the difference between the two word and compound values differences and dividing by a subject's mean f_o in sentences to normalize for mean f_o differences between subjects.

(11) To measure f_o changes in sentence intonation, the high (H) and low (L) points on the intonation curve were measured as indicated in the following sentence:

(F) Say (L)   (L)that's(H)   (L)ex(H)cellent(L)

Five differences between adjacent low and high f_o points were averaged and divided by the subject's mean f_o in sentences to normalize for mean f_o differences between subjects.

(12)   The range of f_o on imitation of an ascending pitch glide was divided by the subject's mean f_o in sentences to normalize for f_o differences between subjects.

(13)   Six measures were made of period length and period amplitude
changes from extended phonation of the vowel /ɑ/ following
analog and digital signal processing. Minor filtering of the speech
waveform insured exponential decay following the point of glottal
excitation. A peak detector circuit eliminated the need for extensive inverse filtering and produced sharp rises at the beginning of
each pitch period. The distances between sharp rises in the peak
detector circuit output waveform were measured using conventional zero crossing techniques.

For each period, voltages were then generated (i) proportional to
the distances between each successive transitions to represent
period length and (ii) proportional to the period amplitude.

The voltage representing period length was converted into hertz
prior to A/D conversion and computer computations. The voltage
representing amplitude was digitized directly and percentage of
variation between adjacent periods was derived. Greater detail on
these analytic procedures is available elsewhere (Ludlow, Coulter,
& Gentges, 1983b). Three indices were computed each from the
frequency and amplitude data.

Mean frequency perturbation (jitter) and *mean amplitude perturbation* (shimmer) were computed by summing the absolute differences in
consecutive period lengths or amplitudes, and dividing by the number of
periods minus one. This dividend was used since, for example, if there
were 10 periods, only nine differences were to be calculated. The mean
frequency perturbation and the mean amplitude perturbation were
calculated over at least 10 blocks, each block containing 50 period
subaverages. Erroneous data was rejected such as frequently occurs at
the beginning and end of each phonation.

It was expected that diplophonia could occur in some patients' phonations due to adjacent periods alternating between two different cycle
lengths or amplitudes. In diplophonia, perturbation computed using
every consecutive period is a great deal larger than when every other
period is used. The degree of diplophonia was measured by dividing the
perturbation using adjacent periods by the perturbation using alternating
periods over each 50 period block. If this ratio became greater than 2.0 it
would indicate the occurrence of diplophonia and is referred to as the
diplophonia ratio (DR).

To assess the slow systematic changes in frequency and amplitude over
several cycles, a measure of deviation from linear trend was computed by

the following formula which was then subtracted from the total perturbation when both were computed using alternating periods (see Ludlow
et al., 1983b). The resulting measure was termed *Linear Trend* (LT) and
contained only slow, systematic variations in frequency or amplitude.

$$\text{Deviation From Linear Trend} = \frac{X_1 - X_5}{2} - X_3$$

Linear Trend = (Mean Perturbation) − (Deviation From Linear Trend)

From these 13 acoustic analyses, 28 acoustic measures resulted. The
names and definitions of these are presented in Appendix 6-B.

Results

The acoustic and perceptual variables could both be subgrouped into
the same six measurement categories: Rate Control, F_o/Pitch Control,
Intensity/Loudness Control, Stress Control, Articulation and Voicing
Control, and Voice Quality. Therefore, our purpose was to examine only
perceptual and acoustic variables within the same measurement category
for inter-relationships. The perceptual system ratings were based on
degree of deviance from normal. For the acoustic measures to also reflect
the degree of deviation from normal, Z scores were computed for each
patient on each variable by the following formula, using the mean and
standard deviation values for the normal control group on the same
variable.

$$Z = \frac{\text{Subject's value–Normal Mean}}{\text{Normal Standard Deviation}}$$

Thus, the degree of deviation from normal for each patient on each
measure was reflected by Z-score values. In the following tables, the
means and standard deviations for each acoustic variable are reported
for each group as well as the mean Z scores and the range in Z scores for
the patients on the acoustic variables. The mean and standard deviations
of the perceptual ratings for the patients and controls are also presented
within each of 6 measurement categories. The inter-relationships between these acoustic and perceptual variables within the patients were
determined using Z scores representing patients' performances on each
acoustic variable and their mean ratings on each perceptual variable
within a measurement category.

TABLE 6-1
Mean and standard deviations of 12 hypokinetic Parkinson patients and 12 age- and sex-matched normal controls on acoustic measures of rate control.

Acoustic Measure	PATIENT GROUP		CONTROL GROUP		PATIENT Z SCORES		% patients with Z of p ≤ .10
	Mean	SD	Mean	SD	Group Mean	Range	
Time of regular rate of sentence production (secs)	3.7	0.5	3.8	0.6	-0.24	-1.70 to +1.40	10[a]
Time of fast rate of sentence production (secs)	2.8	0.4	2.5	0.5	0.59	-0.50 to +1.70	30[a]
Difference in time between regular and fast rates	0.9	0.4	1.3	0.4	-1.10	-2.70 to +0.30	50[a]
Increasing rate on CV syllable repetition (per 5 secs)	-0.7	1.3	-0.6	0.4	-0.17	-8.50 to +2.75	25
Latency of /a/ initiation (secs)	0.5	0.3	0.4	0.1	1.03	-1.32 to +9.00	33

[a]Pro-rated on 10 subjects due to incorrect imitation of sentences for two subjects.

Rate Control

The mean and standard deviations of the patients and controls on the 5 acoustic measures of rate and the 5 perceptual rating categories are presented in Tables 6-1 and 6-2 respectively. In the far right column of Table 6-1 the percentage of the patient group with Z scores in the impaired direction reflecting an acoustic measure outside of the range of 90% of the normal subjects is presented. From these data the relative degree of impairment can be determined for the hypokinetic subjects on the acoustic measures of rate control.

Based on previous descriptions of accelerating rate in hypokinetic patients, the time of regular sentence production was expected to be reduced below normal, yielding Z scores of -1.3 or less in many of the patients. However, an examination of the patients' data indicated that only one patient had an excessively fast rate, while another had an excessively slow rate ($Z = \pm 1.3$, $p = .10$). Therefore, as a group the patients did not differ from normal in their rate of sentence production. On the fast rate of sentence production, three of the patients had an abnormally slow rate, that is, their time of fast sentence production was greater than normal. The difference in time between the regular and fast rates, however, was reduced below the normal range in half of the patients, indicating that a reduced ability to alter speech rate was a characteristic of the hypokinetic group.

TABLE 6-2
Mean and standard deviations for 12 hypokinetic Parkinson patients and 12 age- and sex-matched normal controls on perceptual ratings of rate control.

Rating Category	PATIENT GROUP		CONTROL GROUP		% of Patients with rating ≥ 3
	Mean	SD	Mean	SD	
Overall rate	7.4	1.8	7.5	1.6	17[a]
Increasing rate	2.1	0.6	1.8	0.5	8
Inappropriate silence	3.1	1.7	1.9	1.1	50
Variable rate	3.8	1.1	2.8	1.2	83
Short rushes	1.0	0.0	1.0	0.0	0

[a]Based on a 13-point scale, % of patients rated as having an increasing rate (rating ≥ 10).

Another measure of increasing rate was the change in rate of syllable production during rapid repetition of the same syllable for seven seconds. When the number repeated in the first 1.5 sec was subtracted from those produced in the last 1.5 sec, a positive number would indicate an increasing rate of repetition. An increasing rate greater than 90% of the normal population was found in 3 subjects. However, the reverse was true in three other patients who had rates decreasing to a greater degree than estimated in 90% of normals. Thus, a tendency for an increasing rate or a decreasing rate was not found in the patient group as whole.

Finally, the latency of phonatory initiation was examined to determine whether patients had difficulties with speech initiation following an external signal. Here, 4 of the 12 patients had latencies longer than estimated for 90% of normals. Two of these were the oldest patients, 73 and 70 years old, with one having a latency similar to her age-matched normal control. Thus only two patients had latencies which were abnormal for their age, and phonatory initiation problems were not notable for the group as a whole.

Table 6-2 presents the mean perceptual ratings for the patients and their controls. Since a rating of 3 indicated that a patient presented with a mild impairment more than 75% of the time, the percentage of the patient group with ratings of 3 or greater is presented in the far right column. Overall rate was judged on a 13-point scale, with 7 representing normal. Only 17% of the patients were judged to have an excessively rapid rate and only one (8%) was found to have an increasing rate. None of the subjects exhibited short rushes.

Therefore, the perceptual ratings were similar to the acoustic measures in not finding problems with a rapid and increasing speech rate similar to those reported elsewhere (Darley et al., 1969). The perceptual rating of a variable rate, however, was found in 83% of the patients. Thus, the subjects were judged unable to control their speech rate according to the demands of the tasks presented. There are two possible reasons for this discrepancy between our results and those of Darley et al. (1969). Perhaps, speech imitation or production tasks do not elicit this symptom, while oral reading and conversational speech do. Another explanation may be the advances in medications for patients with Parkinson's disease over the last decade (Calne, 1977). Darley et al. (1969) used tape recordings of patients gathered during the 1960s. At that time, effective levels of medication were not well developed. On the other hand, the patients in this investigation were all receiving medication at levels found to be maximally effective for them. Such medications are now so effective that patients cannot be found off medication, except immediately after diagnosis of the disease. Therefore, differences between our findings and previous findings of others on similar tasks may be attributable to advances in treatment for the disease. It is interesting to note that one of the problems with levodopa and particularly with bromocriptine, is the drug-induced dyskinesia that appears at high dosages in Parkinson patients (Chase, Holden, & Brody, 1973). Although we included patients who exhibited only hypokinesia during testing and who had no apparent dyskinetic movements, the speech symptoms of patients receiving effective treatment may become more similar to patients with dyskinesia, a hyperkinetic dysarthria. If this were the case, it is relevant that variable rate was found by Darley et al. (1969) to be a major characteristic of hyperkinetic dysarthria in chorea, while short rushes of speech was not a feature in chorea.

TABLE 6-3
Pearson Correlation Coefficients between hypokinetic patient Z scores on acoustic measures and perceptual ratings assessing rate control.

| | PERCEPTUAL RATING CATEGORIES | | | |
Acoustic Measure	Overall Rate	Increasing Rate	Inappropriate Silence	Variable Rate
Time of regular rate of sentence production	-.84*	-.03	-.23	-.13
Time of fast rate of sentence production	-.77*	.04	.21	.17
Difference in time between regular and fast rates	-.41	-.07	-.50	-.33
Increasing rate on CV syllable repetition	.45	-.26	.22	-.33
Latency of /ɑ/ initiation	.39	-.12	.77**	.31

* $p \leq .01$, $df = 10$.
**$p \leq .01$, $df = 12$.

Table 6-3 presents the Pearson correlation coefficients between the acoustic measures and perceptual ratings of rate control in the hypokinetic patients. Three significant ($p \leq .01$) relationships were found. Subjects rated as having fast rates produced sentences in less time both at regular rate and fast speaking rates. Further, subjects with longer latencies for phonation initiation were those judged to have greater inappropriate silences. Therefore, these speech tasks provided valid measures of two perceptual dimensions, speech rate and inappropriate silences. However, the acoustic rate measure that was most impaired in the patients (change in sentence rate), did not relate to any of the perceptual ratings and may represent an inability of subjects to modify their speech rate. This aspect was not assessed by the perceptual system of Darley et al. (1969).

Pitch and Fundamental Frequency (f_o) Control

Table 6-4 presents the mean and standard deviations of the f_o acoustic measures for the two groups. The mean fundamental frequency in sentences was higher than that of the age- and sex-matched controls. This is contrary to the pitch judgments of Darley et al. (1969), who found hypokinetic patients had an excessively low pitch. Due to large differences in f_o between males and females, group comparisons are not appropriate on this measure. Rather each patient should be evaluated in comparison with his or her normal control. Eleven of the patients had higher f_o values than their age- and sex-matched normal controls. Therefore, our findings are more in agreement with those of Canter (1963), who found a higher median frequency than normal in patients with Parkinson's disease.

The second measure of maximum range in f_o on the pitch glide task demonstrated that the f_o range was limited in 75% of the patients to a greater degree than in 90% of the normal population. Similar reductions in f_o change were measured on imitation of sentence intonation patterns (7 patients were impaired) and on the use of f_o change to contrast compound nouns with two equally stressed words (impaired in 5 patients).

Table 6-5 presents the perceptual ratings for overall pitch. Six patients had impaired ratings on this; three were judged abnormally high and three were judged abnormally low. Eight of the 12 patients had ratings higher than their controls. Therefore, we failed to replicate the results of Darley et al. (1969) on pitch level ratings as well as the acoustic f_o measures. This may have been due to measurement technique. Canter (1963) also used acoustic methods to measure f_o and found it higher than in normal controls. The improved medications for our patients may have also had an effect. We have observed, as have others, that the vocal folds of severely hypokinetic Parkinson patients are excessively bowed (Ward, Hanson, & Berci, 1981a; 1981b). The patients with less rigidity due to medication may achieve better closure and, hence, a higher f_o. The monopitch ratings were abnormal as were the severity of pitch breaks in 8 of the patients. The first finding is similar to Darley et al. (1969) and others (Canter 1963) while the second was not found to be characteristic of any of the patient groups studied by Darley et al. (1969). This discrepancy may be due, in part, to task differences between the two studies. The perceptual ratings in our study were based on patient's imitation of intonation patterns while the Darley et al. (1969) ratings were made from oral reading and conversational speech.

Table 6-6 presents the correlation coefficients between the acoustic and perceptual measures of pitch/f_o control. Only two relationships were

TABLE 6-4
Mean and standard deviations of 12 hypokinetic Parkinson patients and 12 age- and sex-matched normal controls on acoustic measures of fundamental frequency control for speech.

Acoustic Measure	PATIENT GROUP		CONTROL GROUP		PATIENT Z SCORES		% patients with Z of $p \leq .10$
	Mean	SD	Mean	SD	Group Mean	Range	
Average f_o in sentences (Hz),	165.80	40.70	143.30	38.60	0.58	-0.8 to +2.3	NA[a]
f_o Range (Hz/mean f_o)	0.77	0.30	1.58	0.51	-1.66	-2.6 to +0.8	75
f_o Change in sentence (Hz/mean f_o)	0.30	0.11	0.60	0.21	-1.52	-2.5 to -0.5	58
f_o Change for stress contrasts (Hz/mean f_o)							
Sentence C	0.18	0.14	0.38	0.17	-1.12	-2.4 to -0.0	42
Sentence E	0.18	0.15	0.34	0.24	-0.58	-1.9 to +1.0	17

[a]Not appropriate due to the large differences between male and female f_o values.

TABLE 6-5
Mean and standard deviations for 12 hypokinetic Parkinson patients and 12 age- and sex-matched normal controls on perceptual ratings of pitch.

Rating Category	PATIENT GROUP		CONTROL GROUP		% of Patients with rating ≥ 3
	Mean	*SD*	*Mean*	*SD*	
Pitch Level	6.9	2.3	5.0	1.6	25[a]
Monopitch	3.7	1.2	1.9	0.6	67
Pitch breaks (Uncontrolled pitch variation)	3.7	1.2	3.9	0.7	67

[a]Based on a 13-point scale, % of patients rated as having lowered pitch level (rating ≤ 4).

statistically significant. Those patients with a reduced f_o range on the pitch glide task were those judged to exhibit monopitch to the greatest degree. The other relationship indicated that those using a high f_o were judged to have more uncontrolled pitch breaks. In summary then, the pitch glide task measuring range in f_o was found to be a valid measure of monopitch, a particular characteristic of hypokinetic dysarthria.

TABLE 6-6
Pearson Correlation Coefficients between hypokinetic patient Z scores on acoustic measures of fundamental frequency control and perceptual ratings assessing pitch control.

Acoustic Measure	PERCEPTUAL RATING CATEGORIES		
	Pitch Level	*Monopitch*	*Pitch Breaks*
Average f_o in sentences	.24	-.11	.50*
f_o Range	-.03	-.65**	-.33
f_o Change in sentences	.11	-.10	-.20
f_o Change for stress contrasts			
Sentence C	.42	.32	.14
Sentence E	.31	-.07	.21

*$p \leq .05$, df = 12.
**$p \leq .01$, df = 12.

TABLE 6-7
Mean and standard deviations of 12 hypokinetic Parkinson patients and 12 age- and sex-matched normal controls on acoustic measures of intensity control during speech production.

Acoustic Measure	PATIENT GROUP		CONTROL GROUP		PATIENT Z SCORES		% patients with Z of p ≤ .10
	Mean	SD	Mean	SD	Group Mean	Range	
Average intensity in sentences (dB SPL re .0002 dynes/cm²)	75.9	9.6	78.6	3.1	-0.87	-7.6 to +4.3	42
Intensity range (dB SPL re .0002 dynes/cm)	18.1	4.6	25.6	4.7	-1.60	-3.3 to -1.4	58
Extended phonation length (secs.)	23.9	10.2	35.9	11.5	-1.04	-2.3 to +0.4	33

Loudness and Intensity Control

Table 6-7 presents the results of three measures of the intensity control for speech; average speaking intensity, maximum range in intensity and length of extended phonation. Seven of the 12 patients (or 58%) were reduced in their maximum range of intensity below the range of 90% of the normals. This was not due to the group as a whole having reduced speech intensity. On average intensity in sentences, five subjects had Z scores below 90% of the normals while two had Z scores above 95% of normal subjects. In these latter two patients, restriction in intensity range may be the result of too great an intensity in regular speech. Thus, we did not find a reduction in intensity similar to Canter (1963) although we did find a reduced range in intensity in the majority of the patients.

Table 6-8 presents the results of the perceptual ratings for the subjects. Similar results were found to those in the corresponding acoustic measures. Forty-two percent, (5 patients) had excessively softer voices than normal, while one patient's voice was excessively loud. Monoloudness was found in 58% (7 of the patients) and therefore yielded similar information to our acoustic results and previously reported findings by Darley et al. (1969).

TABLE 6-8
Mean and standard deviations for 12 hypokinetic Parkinson patients and 12 age- and sex-matched normal controls on perceptual ratings of loudness control.

Rating Category	PATIENT GROUP		CONTROL GROUP		% of Patients with rating ≥ 3
	Mean	*SD*	*Mean*	*SD*	
Overall loudness	6.1	2.7	8.8	1.7	42[a]
Uncontrolled loudness variation	3.6	1.4	2.4	0.4	58
Monoloudness	3.7	1.4	2.7	1.0	67

[a]Based on a 13-point scale, % of patients rated as having decreased loudness rate (rating ≤ 4).

Table 6-9 presents the Pearson correlation coefficients between the two sets of measures. The results indicate that the task to produce different loudness levels and acoustic measurement of the intensity levels achieved is a valid procedure for determining subjects' intensity variation for speech.

TABLE 6-9

Pearson Correlation Coefficients between hypokinetic patient Z scores on acoustic measures of intensity and perceptual ratings assessing loudness control.

	PERCEPTUAL RATING CATEGORIES		
Acoustic Measure	Overall Loudness	Uncontrolled Loudness Variation	Monoloudness
Average Intensity in sentences	.36	-.39	-.43
Intensity Range	.41	-.18	-.67**
Extended Phonation Length	.43	-.50*	-.49*

*$p \leq .05$, $df = 12$.
**$p \leq .01$, $df = 12$.

Stress-Timing Control

Three acoustic measures were made from spectrographs of the timing contrasts used by subjects to mark word boundaries to differentiate two nouns as separate from two nouns as a compound. The time between initiation of the two words in each condition was determined and the differences in time between the two conditions computed. Based on previous reports of an increasing rate and fast speech rate in Parkinson's disease, we expected word boundaries would be less distinct and that the pause length would be reduced in the two noun conditions with less of a difference between the compound and two-word conditions. Table 6-10 presents the results that indicate 58% (7 of the patients) had reduced differences in word boundary lengths between the two conditions which were less than those of 90% of the normal distribution. However this difference was not because the patients had markedly reduced word lengths in either condition. Only 33% (4 patients) had word lengths shorter than those of 90% of the normals. Therefore, the patients were unable to alter their rate of speech production at the word length level, but were within normal limits in their usual rate of production of both separate nouns and compound nouns. Table 6-11 presents the perceptual ratings for reduced stress and excess stress. Reduced stress was judged impaired in only 33% of the patients. Thus, stress was not as impaired in our patients as would have been expected from the Darley et al. (1969) results who found this the second most salient characteristic in hypokinetic dysarthria.

TABLE 6-10
Mean and standard deviations of 12 hypokinetic Parkinson patients and 12 age- and sex-matched normal controls on acoustic measures of stress-timing control for speech.

Acoustic Measure	PATIENT GROUP		CONTROL GROUP		PATIENT Z SCORES		% patients with Z of p ≤ .10
	Mean	SD	Mean	SD	Group Mean	Range	
Interword interval length (sec)	0.94	0.21	1.16	0.25	-0.88	-1.7 to +0.4	33
Intersyllable interval length (sec)	0.53	0.09	0.50	0.07	0.29	-1.2 to +1.9	17
Change in interval length to achieve linguistic contrast (sec)	0.41	0.23	0.67	0.23	-1.46	-2.5 to +1.0	58

TABLE 6-11
Mean and standard deviations for 12 hypokinetic Parkinson patients and 12 age- and sex-matched normal controls on perceptual ratings of stress control.

Rating Category	PATIENT GROUP		CONTROL GROUP		% of Patients with
	Mean	SD	Mean	SD	rating ≤ 3
Reduced stress	2.8	1.3	1.6	1.2	33
Excess stress	1.1	0.3	1.1	0.3	0

Table 6-12 presents the Pearson correlation coefficients between the acoustic and perceptual measures. The strongest relationsip was between ratings of reduced stress and the interword interval in the two-word condition. Those patients with shorter intervals had the more severe ratings. The relationship between the difference in length between the different word boundary conditions and reduced stress ratings, although statistically significant, was less marked. Thus, interword intervals between two separate nouns and comparison with compound noun intersyllable intervals were valid reflections of reduced stress in the hypokinetic patients studied.

TABLE 6-12
Pearson Correlation Coefficients between hypokinetic patient Z scores on acoustic measures and perceptual ratings assessing stress-timing control.

Acoustic Measure	PERCEPTUAL RATING CATEGORIES	
	Reduced Stress	Excess Stress
Interword interval length	-.75**	.56*
Intersyllable interval length	-.26	.21
Change in interval length to achieve linguistic contrast	-.59*	.44

*$p \leq .05$, $df = 12$.
**$p \leq .01$, $df = 12$.

Voicing Control and Articulation

The results of the acoustic measures of voicing control and the coordination of phonatory onset and offset with speech articulation are presented in Table 6-13. The number of on-off phonations during vowel repetition measured the ability of subjects to rapidly onset and offset

TABLE 6-13

Mean and standard deviations of 12 hypokinetic Parkinson patients and 12 age- and sex-matched normal controls on acoustic measures of articulation and voicing control during speech production.

Acoustic Measure	PATIENT GROUP		CONTROL GROUP		PATIENT Z SCORES			% patients with Z of p ≤.10
	Mean	SD	Mean	SD	Group Mean	SD	Range	
No. of vowel voicing errors per 5 secs	27.7	26.2	2.5	9.1	2.77		-0.6 to +8.4	64*
No. of consonant voicing errors per 5 secs	-0.4	5.1	-3.2	1.7	1.67		-1.1 to +6.6	33*
Voicing differences between tense /i/ vs. lax /ɑ/ vowel syllable repetitions	-0.4	7.8	2.1	5.0	-0.49		-3.4 to +1.6	18**
Voicing differences between tongue blade /k/ vs. tip /t/ CV syllable repetitions	1.3	2.6	0.0	1.7	0.75		-0.6 to +4.7	18**
No. of on-off phonations vowel /ɑ/ repetitions (per 5 secs)	11.0	8.1	20.3	4.0	-2.33		-4.8 to +1.2	73*
No. of on-off phonations for CV syllable /pɑ/ repetitions (per 5 secs)	21.0	5.9	23.0	7.0	-0.29		-2.1 to +1.1	8*

Note. Pro-rated on 11 patients.

*Z ≥-1.3 (1-tailed).

**Z ≥±1.65 (2-tailed).

phonation. The same aspect was measured when there was coordinated valving of the airstream by lip closure preceding the onset and offset of phonation during /pɑ/ repetition. Seventy-three percent (8 of the 11 patients tested) had fewer on-off phonations on vowel repetitions than 90% of normals. The same impairment was not found on stop plosive CV syllable repetition where the number of on-off phonations was within the normal distribution in all but one of the patients. The supralaryngeal valving of the airstream at the lips seemed to assist the patients in achieving rapid onsets and offsets of phonation.

To measure the accuracy of phonatory control for speech articulation, the correspondence between the number of gaps in phonation (on-off phonation) and the number of vowel or syllable repetitions was computed from repetitions of /ɑ/ and from repetition of /pɑ/ and were designated as the number of vowel voicing errors and number of consonantal voicing errors respectively. The number of vowel voicing errors in 64% of the patients was greater than in 90% of normals, while the voicing errors on stop plosive CV syllable repetition was outside the normal distribution in only 33% of the patients. Thus, the coordination of laryngeal and oral gestures did not seem to be particularly impaired in these patients. Rather it was the rapid onset and offset of phonation, when not coordinated with other articulatory gestures, that seemed to present the greatest difficulty.

To measure differences between voicing control on repetitions of tense and lax vowels that have different tongue positions, the number of on-off phonations during /ɑ/ repetition minus the number during /i/ repetition was computed. Only two of the patients were impaired on this measure indicating that tongue position did not influence voicing control in the patients in comparison with normal.

Finally, to measure differences between voicing control on repetitions of tongue blade and tongue tip plosive CV syllables, the number of on-off phonations during /tɑ/ repetition minus the number during /kɑ/ repetition was computed. Here again, the tongue position and point of articulation did not influence voicing control in the hypokinetic patients in comparison with normal.

In Table 6-14, the mean rating for imprecise consonants was abnormal in four subjects. This result is dissimilar to that of Darley et al. (1969) who found this impaired in all of their patients with Parkinson's disease.

Table 6-15 presents the Pearson correlation coefficients between the acoustic measures and the perceptual ratings of imprecise articulatory precision. Two of the acoustic measures reflected ratings of articulation: the number of voicing errors on stop plosive CV syllables and the number of phonatory offsets and onsets on the repetition of /tɑ/ versus

TABLE 6-14
Mean and standard deviations for 12 hypokinetic Parkinson patients and 12 age- and sex-matched normal controls on perceptual ratings of speech articulation.

Rating Category	PATIENT GROUP		CONTROL GROUP		% of Patients with rating ≤ 3
	Mean	*SD*	*Mean*	*SD*	
Imprecise consonants	3.3	1.8	1.7	0.4	33

/kɑ/. Those with voicing errors and those with a greater number of phonatory onsets and offsets on /tɑ/ than on /kɑ/ were judged to have more imprecise articulation. These relationships confirm our impressions that the more impaired subjects had greater substitutions of voiced plosives for unvoiced plosives on /pɑ/ repetitions. Also, in the severely impaired patients, the production of tongue blade consonants was more difficult than tongue tip articulations.

Neither of these measures, however, were those particularly impaired in the hypokinetic patients in Table 6-13. Although poor voicing control for vowels was impaired in the large majority of the patients, this did not seem to contribute to listeners' impressions of poor articulation. The

TABLE 6-15
Pearson Correlation Coefficients between hypokinetic patient Z scores on acoustic measures and perceptual ratings assessing articulation and voicing control.

Acoustic Measure	PERCEPTUAL RATING CATEGORIES *Imprecise Consonants*
No. of vowel voicing errors	-.09
No. of consonant voicing errors	.62*
Voicing Differences Between:	
Tense vs. lax vowel syllable repetitions	-.19
Tongue blade vs. back CV syllable repetitions	.55*
No. of on-off phonations for:	
Vowel repetitions /ɑ/	-.08
CV syllable repetitions /pɑ/	-.50**

*p ≤ .05, df = 11.
**p ≤ .05, df = 12.

TABLE 6-16

Mean and standard deviations of 12 hypokinetic Parkinson patients and 12 age- and sex-matched normal controls on acoustic measures of frequency and intensity perturbation during extended phonation.

Acoustic Measure	PATIENT GROUP		CONTROL GROUP		PATIENT Z SCORES		% patients with Z of p ≤ .10
	Mean	SD	Mean	SD	Group Mean	Range	
Mean frequency perturbation (secs)	43.6	24.9	50.1	15.3	-0.43	-2.8 to + 2.6	17
Frequency diplophonia ratio	1.21	0.34	1.19	0.36	0.05	-1.6 to + 2.0	8
Frequency linear trend	5.9	3.0	7.7	4.1	-0.43	-1.7 to + 1.0	0
Mean intensity perturbation (dB)	7.7	6.1	4.5	1.6	2.06	-1.4 to +10.7	50
Intensity diplophonia ratio	1.05	0.50	0.95	0.27	0.39	-1.7 to + 5.8	8
Intensity linear trend	0.87	0.54	0.60	0.22	1.24	-0.9 to + 8.4	50

most valid measures of indistinct articulation in this patient group were
consonant voicing errors and difficulties with /ka/ repetition.

Voice Quality

Table 6-16 presents the acoustic measures of frequency and intensity
perturbation, diplophonia, and linear trend. Only two of these measures
were impaired in half of the patients: mean intensity perturbation and
linear trend in intensity. Thus, intensity was less controlled in the patients, but not frequency.

Only two of the subjects were outside of the normal range for frequency perturbation. Thus, this attribute was not increased in the phonation
of patients with neurological abnormalities and appears rather to be affected by morphological changes in the larynx (Ludlow et al., 1983a).
The finding that greater than normal intensity perturbation occurred
during sustained phonation may relate to vocal fold position during
phonation in these patients. In several hypokinetic patients, we have
observed a bowing of the vocal folds during phonation as have others
(Ward et al., 1981a, 1981b). This abnormal positioning of the folds may
result in greater airflow turbulence and, therefore, more variation in intensity between periods. The linear trend measure of slow systematic
variations in period intensity, was also excessive in 50% of the patients.
Attempts to alter vocal fold positioning or subglottal pressure during
phonation may account for these slow changes in intensity during phonation in the Parkinson patients.

Table 6-17 presents the results of ratings on six perceptual categories
of voice quality. Harsh voice was found in 10 of the 12 patients,
replicating the findings of Darley et al. (1969). These investigators found

TABLE 6-17
**Mean and standard deviations for 12 hypokinetic Parkinson patients and 12 age- and sex-
matched normal controls on perceptual ratings of voice quality.**

Rating Category	PATIENT GROUP		CONTROL GROUP		% of Patients with rating ≥ 3
	Mean	SD	Mean	SD	
Harsh voice	3.5	1.0	3.9	0.9	83
Hoarse (wet) voice	2.0	1.6	2.2	0.9	33
Hypernasality	2.9	1.8	2.9	0.7	42
Strained-strangled voice	2.3	0.7	1.7	0.6	17
Breathy voice	2.3	1.3	1.4	0.5	17
Glottal fry	1.5	0.6	1.5	0.5	0

harshness and breathinesss to be salient characteristics in hypokinetic dysarthria. We found breathiness was noticable only in two patients. As we indicated earlier, the medications administered to our patients might have made our patients less hypokinetic and closer to hyperkinetic. In this light, Darley et al. (1969) reported high harsh voice ratings for both hypokinetic and hyperkinetic dysarthria, but breathiness only in the hypokinetic group.

Table 6-18 presents the relationships found between the acoustic and perceptual ratings of voice quality. The only significant ($p \leq .01$) positive relationships found were between intensity perturbation and breathiness, and between linear trend in intensity and breathiness. The latter relationship was particularly strong, indicating that linear trend in intensity could account for 70% of the variance in breathiness ratings, and was a good reflection of breathiness in these patients. Also, both intensity perturbation and linear trend in intensity were greater than normal in 50% of the patients. Thus, these acoustic measures may be good indicators of one aspect of phonatory pathology in Parkinson patients, reflecting abnormal variations in intensity possibly caused by problems with airflow through the glottis. However, the perceptual rating most impaired in the patients was harshness, which did not relate to any of the acoustic measures. Measures of the distribution of energy across the frequency

TABLE 6-18
Pearson Correlation Coefficients between hypokinetic patient Z scores on acoustic measures of frequency and intensity perturbation and perceptual ratings assessing voice quality.

| Acoustic Measure | PERCEPTUAL RATING CATEGORIES | | | | | |
	Harsh Voice	Hoarse Voice	Hyper-nasality	Strained-Strangled Voice	Breathy Voice	Glottal Fry
Frequency:						
Mean perturbation	.32	.27	-.76**	.10	.01	-.03
Diplophonia ratio	.10	-.15	-.16	-.12	-.14	.27
Linear trend	.14	-.14	-.16	.34	.08	-.32
Intensity:						
Mean perturbation	.02	.10	.23	-.30	.69**	.20
Diplophonia ratio	.13	-.15	-.13	.22	.02	-.20
Linear trend	.02	-.11	.16	-.59*	.84**	.47

*$p \leq .05$, $df = 12$.
**$p \leq .01$, $df = 12$.

spectrum (Hirano, 1981) may relate to harshness and should be studied in hypokinetic patients.

DISCUSSION AND CONCLUSIONS

The purpose of this study was to determine the validity of a set of objective and quantitative acoustic measures for reflecting those perceptual attributes previously demonstrated to be associated with hypokinetic dysarthria by Darley et al. (1969). Thus, perceptual ratings similar to those used by Darley et al. (1969) were used in this study. As one step in demonstrating that the acoustic measures are valid reflectors of perceptual ratings, it was of interest to determine if our perceptual ratings of Parkinson patients replicated those of Darley et al. (1969). The mean ratings of Darley et al. (1969) and of our three judges on the same attributes are presented in Table 6-19 along with the rank ordering from most severe to least affected attribute within each set of ratings. The differences in rank orders within the two rating scales are presented in the right-hand column.

TABLE 6-19
Comparison of the mean perceptual ratings of this study and those of Darley, Aronson, & Brown (1969) on hypokinetic patients.

| | DARLEY et al. | | THIS STUDY | | DIFFERENCES |
| | *Mean* | | *Mean* | | *IN RANKS* |
Perceptual Categories	*Rating*	*Rank*	*Rating*	*Rank*	
Monopitch	4.64	1	3.71	2	1
Reduced stress	4.46	2	2.78	7	5
Monoloudness	4.26	3	3.66	3	0
Imprecise consonants	3.59	4	3.28	5	1
Inappropriate silences	2.40	5	3.12	6	1
Short rushes	2.22	6	1.00	10	4
Harsh voice	2.08	7	3.48	4	3
Breathy voice	2.04	8	2.33	8	0
Low pitch	1.76	9	1.12	9	0
Variable rate	1.74	10	3.77	1	9

There was good agreement on six of the dimensions. A difference in ranks of three or more occurred on four categories: reduced stress, short rushes, harsh voice, and variable rate. In this study, reduced stress and short rushes were less severe than in the Darley et al. (1969) patients. Conversely, variable rate and harsh voice were more prominent in our patients. These differences indicated that our patients were more similar to patients with hyperkinetic dysarthria such as in chorea or dyskinesia. This may be a result of the administration of the levodopa and/or the use of bromocriptine in most of our patients. Many of these treatments can induce dyskinesia to various degrees in Parkinson patients (Chase et al., 1973). The dosage must be adjusted in patients to achieve the maximum relief from rigidity (which can immobilize a patient almost completely) while at the same time not inducing dyskinesia to the extent that it interferes with the patient's ability to control his other voluntary movement (Godwin-Austen, 1973). All of our patients had undergone careful observation to achieve their maximally effective dosage. Therefore, the administration of dopamine enhancing treatment in Parkinson patients may have changed the characteristics of dysarthria typically seen in such patients. Thus, our patients may have been relieved of their rapid rushes of speech, increasing rate, and reductions in stress with dopamine enhancement therapy. However at the same time, they exhibited more problems controlling their rate from varying sporadically and had a harsher vocal quality than Darley et al. (1969) patients. As pharmacologic treatments are developed for neurologic disease, clinicians should be alert to changes that may occur in the patient's speech and the factors that need to be modified to improve communicative ability.

To return to our major purpose in this investigation, (i.e., to identify acoustic measures of speech function), those measures which relate to perceptual categories and are found to be impaired in hypokinesia are listed in Table 6-20. These measures, therefore, are all recommended for the assessment of the pattern and severity of speech production impairment in Parkinson patients and would be most useful for assessing treatment effects in such patients. The mean Z scores reflect the degree of deviation from normal for the group as a whole. These Z scores are ranked from 1 for most severe to 11 for that least affected in the group. Thus, the ranks indicate the relative degree of impairment of these factors in the dysarthria of patients with Parkinson's disease. The first five factors all reflect laryngeal control: the number of on-off phonations, voicing errors, range in f_o, and range in intensity. Most of the remaining factors reflect rate and stress control: interword interval and the change in interval on stress contrasts, fast speaking rate, latency of initiation, and control of change in rate. Therefore, the acoustic measurement system indicates two dysfunctions as the major contributing factors to speech disturbance in Parkinson's disease. First and foremost was an inability to maneuver speech range. Both of these factors point to these patients' rigidity particularly affecting their ability to maneuver their larynx and articulators to provide the prosodic aspects of speech. Therefore, when

TABLE 6-20
Acoustic measures found to be valid measures of degree of speech impairment in patients with Parkinson's disease.

Acoustic Measure	Mean Z score	Rank Order (1 = Most Severe)	Related Perceptual
Rate of control:			
Time of fast rate	0.59	11	Overall rate
Difference between fast and regular rate	-1.10	8	(None)
Latency of /ɑ/ initiation	1.03	9	Inappropriate silences
F_o Control:			
F_o range on pitch glide	-1.66	3	Monopitch
F_o range in sentences	-1.52	5	(None)
Intensity control:			
Intensity range between soft and shout	-1.60	4	Monoloudness
Stress control:			
Interword interval	-0.88	10	Reduced stress
Change in word length with linguistic contrast	-1.46	6	Reduced stress
Voicing control:			
No. of consonant voicing errors	1.67	2	Imprecise consonants
No. of on-off phona-tions on vowel repetitions	-2.33	1	(None)
Voice quality:			
Linear trend in intensity	1.24	7	Breathiness

assessing the speech of patients with Parkinson's disease we would recommend that Z scores be computed for the 11 acoustic measures found to reflect the degree of a patient's impairment. Such measures should also be useful measures of the efficacy of treatment for improving speech production.

REFERENCES

Calne, D. B. Developments on the pharmacology and therapeutics of Parkinsonsim. *Annals of Neurology,* 1977, *1,* 111-119.

Canter, G. J. Speech characteristics of patients with Parkinson's disease: I. Intensity, pitch, and duration. *Journal of Speech and Hearing Disorders,* 1963, *28,* 221-229.

Canter, G. J. Speech characteristics of patients with Parkinson's disease: II. Physiological Support for Speech. *Journal of Speech and Hearing Disorders,* 1965, *30,* 44-49. (a)

Canter, G. J. Speech characteristics of patients with Parkinson's disease: III. Articulation, Diadochokinesis, and Overall Speech Adequacy. *Journal of Speech and Hearing Disorders,* 1965, *30,* 217-224. (b)

Chase, T. N., Holden, E. M., & Brody, J. A. Levodopa-induced dyskinesias: Comparison in Parkinsonism-dementia and amyotrophic lateral sclerosis. *Archives of Neurology,* 1973, *29,* 328-330.

Darley, F. L., Aronson, A. E., & Brown, J. R. Differential diagnostic patterns of dysarthria. *Journal of Speech and Hearing Research,* 1969, *12,* 246-269.

Godwin-Austen, R. B. The long-term therapeutic effects of levodopa in the treatment of Parkinsonism. *Advances in Neurology,* 1973, *3,* 23-27.

Henderson, W. G., Sandowsky, D. A., Shapiro, D. Y., & Van Buren, J. M. Quantitative testing and its usefulness in the evaluation of therapy in neurological diseases. *Confinia Neurologica,* 1973, *35,* 321-327.

Hirano, M. Clinical examination of voice. In G. E. Arnold, F. Winckel, & B. D. Wyke (Eds.), *Disorders of human communication 5.* New York: Springer-Verlag Wien, 1981.

Lehiste, I. Some acoustic characteristics of dysarthric speech. *Bibliotheca Phonetica, Fasciculus 2.* Basel: Karger, 1965. Vol. 2, pp. 1-124.

Ludlow, C. L., & Bassich, C. J. The results of acoustic and perceptual assessment of two types of dysarthria. In W. R. Berry (Ed.), *Clinical dysarthria.* San Diego: College-Hill Press, 1983, 121-154.

Ludlow, C. L., Coulter, D. C., & Gentges, F. H. The differential sensitivity of frequency perturbation to laryngeal neoplasms and neuropathologies. In D. Bless & J. Abbs (Eds.), *Vocal fold physiology.* San Diego: College-Hill Press 1983. (a)

Ludlow, C. L., Coulter, D. C. & Gentges, F. H. The effects of change in vocal fold morphology on phonation. *Proceedings of the Juilliard Eleventh Symposium: Care of the professional voice,* New York: The Voice Foundation, 1983. (b)

Ward, P. H., Hanson, D. G., & Berci, G. Observations on central neurologic etiology for laryngeal dysfunction. *Annals of Otolaryngology,* 1981, *90,* 430-441. (a)

Ward, P. H., Hanson, D. G. & Berci, G. Photographic studies of the larynx in central laryngeal paresis and paralysis. *Acta Otolaryngology,* 1981, *91,* 353-367. (b)

APPENDIX 6-A:
DEFINITIONS OF PERCEPTUAL RATING CATEGORIES

Name of Attribute	Definition of Attribute
Rate Control:	
Overall rate	Rate of speech is abnormally slow or too rapid.
Increasing rate	Rate becomes increasingly fast within connected speech.
Short rushes	There are short rushes of speech separated by pauses.
Inappropriate silences	There are inappropriate silent intervals.
Variable rate	Rate alternates between slow and fast.
Pitch Control:	
Pitch level	Pitch of voice sounds consistently too low or too high for individual's age and sex.
Pitch breaks (uncontrolled pitch variation)	Pitch of the voice shows sudden, uncontrolled variation (falsetto breaks) or waver and modulation of pitch.
Monopitch	Voice lacks normal pitch and inflectional changes.
Intensity Control:	
Overall loudness	Loudness is either too low or too high in relation to a constant reference signal.
Uncontrolled loudness variation	Voice shows sudden, uncontrolled alterations in loudness, sometimes becoming too loud or too weak.
Monoloudness	Voice lacks normal variations in loudness.
Stress Control:	
Reduced stress	Speech shows reduction of proper stress on emphasis patterns.
Excess stress	There is excess stress on usually unstressed parts of speech.
Voicing Control:	
Imprecise consonants	Consonant sounds are slurred, distorted, lack crispness, and run into each other.
Voice Quality:	
Hypernasality	Voice is excessively nasal. Excessive amount of air is resonated by nasal cavities.
Hoarse voice (wet)	There is wet, liquid-sounding hoarseness.
Glottal fry (diplophonia)	There is bubbly, crackling low-pitched phonation.
Strained-strangled voice	Voice sounds like an effortful squeezing of voice through the glottis.

Breathy voice	Breathy, weak, thin.
Harsh voice	Voice is harsh, rough, and raspy.

APPENDIX 6-B:
DEFINITION OF ACOUSTIC MEASURES

Name of Measure	*Definition of Measure*
Rate Control:	
Regular rate sentence production	Total time for sentence production at regular rate.
Fast rate sentence production	Total time for sentence production at fast rate.
Difference in sentence rate	Time for sentence production at regular rate minus time at fast rate.
Increase in rate on CV syllable repetition	No. of syllables in last 1.5 sec minus no. of syllables in first 1.5 sec during syllable repetitions of 5.5 sec.
Latency of /ɑ/ initiation	Msec between click initiation and onset of phonation.
Fundamental Frequency (f_o) Control:	
Average f_o in sentences	Average of peak f_o on six nouns in three sentences.
f_o range	Difference in Hz between low and high points of an ascending vowel production divided by mean f_o in sentences.
f_o change in sentences	Average of high and low f_o differences in sentence intonation contour divided by mean f_o in sentences.
f_o change in stress	Difference in peak f_o between two words of equal stress minus difference in peak f_o between words of unequal stress, divided by mean f_o in sentences. (C) is the f_o change for the words *blue bell* vs. *bluebell*, (E) is the f_o change for the words *cross word* vs. *crossword*.
Intensity Control:	
Average intensity in sentences	Average of peak sound pressure level on final word of six sentences.
Intensity range	Difference between peak sound pressure level on *shout* production minus that on *soft* production.
Extended phonation length	Length in seconds of extended vowel production at comfortable intensity and f_o.
Stress Control:	
Interword interval length	Difference between initiation of equally stressed nouns.
Intersyllable interval length	Difference between initiation of syllables in compound nouns.

| Change in interval length achieve contrast | Difference between interval for initiation of equally stressed nouns minus interval between initiation times of syllables in compound nouns. |

Voicing Control:

Vowel voicing errors	The number of vowel repetitions minus the number of on-off phonations.
Consonant voicing errors	The number of syllable repetitions minus the number of on-off phonations.
Voicing differences on lax vs. tense vowel repetitions	Number of voicing offsets with /ɑ/ minus number of voicing offsets with /i/.
Voicing differences between /k/ and /t/ CV syllable repetitions	Number of voicing offsets with /kɑ/ repetition minus numbers of voicing offsets with /tɑ/ repetition.
On-off rate /ɑ/	Number of voicing offsets on /ɑ/ repetition.
On-off rate /pɑ/	Number of voicing offsets on /pɑ/ repetition.

Voice Quality:

Mean frequency perturbation (jitter)	Mean perturbation in fundamental freqency (f_o) divided by f_o during extended phonation.
Frequency diplophonia ratio	Mean perturbation for adjacent periods divided by mean perturbation for alternate periods.
Frequency linear trend	Amount of slow systematic change in period length.
Mean intensity perturbation (shimmer)	Mean amplitude variation between periods during extended phonation.
Intensity diplophonia ratio	Mean amplitude variation between adjacent periods divided by mean amplitude variation for alternate periods.
Intensity linear trend	Amount of slow systematic change in period amplitude.

7

Relationships between Articulation Rate, Intelligibility, and Naturalness in Spastic and Ataxic Speakers

Craig W. Linebaugh
Victoria E. Wolfe

INTRODUCTION

An alteration in rate of speech is among the most common signs observed in dysarthric speakers. Of the 212 dysarthric patients examined by Darley, Aronson, and Brown (1969), 170 presented some degree of deviation from normal in their rate of speech. Of these, nearly all presented a reduction in speaking rate, with only hypokinetic dysarthric patients as a group displaying a slightly faster than normal rate.

Reduced speaking rate may reflect a decrease in articulation rate, an increase in intra- and interword pause time, or a combination of the two. There is evidence that, for many dysarthric speakers, their impaired neuromuscular efficiency results in reduced articulation rate (i.e., a slowing of the movement of the articulators during speech). In their extensive perceptual study of seven types of dysarthria, Darley et al. (1969) observed prolongation of individual phonemes in a majority of their spastic, ALS, ataxic, dystonic, and choreatic subjects. Acoustic and physiological evidence of reduced articulation rate in dysarthria has also been obtained. Kent and his colleagues (Kent & Netsell, & Bauer, 1975) have reported longer than normal durations for individual phonetic seg-

ments in the speech of dysarthric individuals. In addition, using cineradiography, they observed markedly slower rates of articulatory movement in several dysarthric speakers. For example, one of their subjects
took three times longer than a normal speaker to move his tongue from
/g/ to /æ/ (Kent et al., 1975).

The purpose of this study was to compare readily obtained, clinically
useful estimates of articulation rate among groups of normal, spastic
dysarthric, and ataxic dysarthric speakers. In addition, we sought to determine the relationships between articulation rate and the overall parameters of intelligibility and naturalness.

METHOD

Subjects

The subjects for this study were 14 spastic dysarthric, 14 ataxic dysarthric, and 14 normal speakers. The mean ages of the spastic dysarthric,
ataxic dysarthric, and normal groups were 57.7, 57.8, and 56.9 years, respectively. The normal-speaking subjects were free of known
neurological impairment. Placement of the dysarthric speakers in the
spastic and ataxic groups was based on a review of their medical histories
and examinations, plus audio-taped samples of their speech production
by a neurologist and two speech-language pathologists as part of a
separate study (Portnoy & Aronson, 1982).

Procedures

Articulation rate. The measure of articulation rate used in this study
was mean syllable duration. Mean syllable duration for each subject was
determined by dividing audible speech emission time by the number of
syllables produced during a reading of the Grandfather Passage. Recorded readings of this passage were randomly selected from a larger sample
used in a recent study by Portnoy and Aronson (1982). All of the recorded readings were free of vocal (e.g., cough, throat clearing) or other
audible artifacts. It is important to note that audible speech emission
time is only an estimate of total articulation time. Nonaudible articulatory movements such as the occlusive phase of plosive consonants
are not included in this measure. However, it may be considered a valid
comparative measure of articulation rate and is more readily obtained
than more inclusive measures (e.g., cineradiography, ultrasound).

To obtain audible speech emission time, each recorded passage was
played back on a Sony TC-353d tape recorder, with output passed
through a Grason-Stadler 1701 audiometer to insure consistent intensity
levels. The output of the audiometer was sent to an array of Coulbourn

Instruments logic modules (see Figure 7-1). Detection of the speech signal was accomplished using a S21-06 bipolar comparator. The threshold for detection of the speech signal was determined by first finding the maximum intensity level at which the bipolar comparator responded to the "noise" on a silent portion of the tape containing the speech samples. The threshold adjustment of the bipolar comparator was then set at 6dB above that level. This threshold level yielded a reliable response to speech signals, while eliminating any recording artifacts. The output of the bipolar comparator was then passed to an S52-12 retriggerable one-shot with 40 msec jumper in place, activating, in turn, a S53-21 universal timer. The audible speech emission time for each speech sample was displayed on an R11-25 electronic counter.

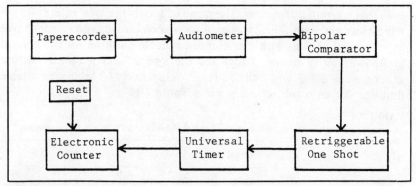

FIGURE 7-1
Schematic diagram of instrumentation used for the measurement of audible speech emission time.

Syllable count. One of the investigators (VEW) listened to each of the recorded passages and used a hand counter to compute the number of syllables produced by the subject.

Intelligibility and naturalness. Ratings of the intelligibility and naturalness of each subject's speech were done on 7-point equal interval scales by five certified speech-language pathologists. A 7 on the scales indicated 100% intelligibility and normal, respectively. The remaining 6 points on the scales were not labeled. The ratings were done in a sound-treated booth. The recorded reading passages were played back on a Sony TC-353d tape recorder, passed through a Grason-Stadler 1701 audiometer, and presented free-field to the raters at a comfortable listening level.

RESULTS

Reliability

To insure the reliability of the syllable counts, a second judge not otherwise involved in the study counted the number of syllables produced by five randomly selected subjects from each of the three subject groups. The discrepancy between the two judges' counts ranged from 0 to 9% of the first judge's counts. The mean discrepancies for the normal, spastic dysarthric, and ataxic dysarthric groups were 1%, 4%, and 3%, respectively.

Interjudge reliability for the intelligibility and naturalness ratings was assessed by intraclass correlations (Winer, 1971). The intraclass correlation for intelligibility was .95. Correlation for naturalness was .93.

Between group differences. The mean of the five judges' ratings for intelligibility and naturalness was used for all comparisons among the three experimental groups. The overall mean syllable duration for the normal group was 197.9 msecs. Those for the spastic and ataxic dysarthric groups were 246.3 and 248.5 msecs., respectively. The mean syllable duration for each subject is shown in Table 7-1.

TABLE 7-1
Mean syllable durations (in milliseconds) for individual subjects in the three groups.

Subject	Normal	Spastic	Ataxic
1	178.6	202.1	263.7
2	194.1	291.6	315.3
3	171.1	250.8	213.8
4	184.7	301.1	242.9
5	208.8	214.1	229.7
6	218.8	266.3	412.5
7	207.6	253.9	235.2
8	209.5	215.2	263.3
9	189.5	216.4	280.1
10	186.4	327.9	269.8
11	200.8	232.7	234.9
12	233.9	221.5	169.3
13	186.2	217.7	255.3
14	209.6	296.1	251.1
$\bar{X}$	197.9	246.3	248.5

The overall mean intelligibility rating for the normal group was 6.9, that for the spastic dysarthric group was 5.9; and mean intelligibility for the ataxic dysarthric group was 5.7. The overall mean naturalness ratings for the normal and spastic and ataxic dysarthric groups were 6.7, 4.5, and 4.2, respectively. Mean intelligibility and naturalness ratings for each subject are shown in Table 7-2..

Pair-wise comparisons of the mean syllable durations, intelligibility ratings, and naturalness ratings for the three groups were made using Mann-Whitney U tests (Siegel, 1956). Nonparametric statistical procedures were used for all the analyses carried out because of the skewed nature of the distributions. The overall mean syllable duration of the normal group was significantly shorter than that of both the spastic dysarthric ($U = 16$, $p < .001$) and the ataxic dysarthric ($U = 10$, $p < .001$) groups. The overall mean syllable durations for the spastic and ataxic dysarthric groups were not significantly different.

The overall mean intelligibility rating of the normal group was significantly higher than those of both the spastic dysarthric group ($U = 2$, $p < .001$) and the ataxic dysarthric group ($U = 0$, $p < .001$). Similarly, the overall mean naturalness rating of the normal group was significantly higher than those of both the spastic ($U = 5$, $p < .001$) and ataxic ($U = 2$, $p < .001$) dysarthric groups. The overall mean ratings of intelligibility and naturalness were not significantly different between the two dysarthric groups.

Correlations Between Mean Syllable Duration and Intelligibility and Naturalness

Spearman Rank Correlation Coefficients (Siegel, 1956) were derived to determine if significant relationships existed between mean syllable duration and intelligibility and naturalness. For the spastic dysarthric group, the correlation between mean syllable duration and intelligibility was significant ($r = -.47$, $p < .05$). Likewise, the correlation of mean syllable duration with naturalness was significant ($r = -.64$, $p < .01$). These findings indicate that as mean syllable duration increased, both intelligibility and naturalness decreased. For the ataxic dysarthric group, the correlation of mean syllable duration with neither intelligibility nor naturalness was significant. The correlations between mean syllable duration and intelligibility and naturalness were not derived for the normal speakers because of the limited range of intelligibility and naturalness ratings for this group.

DISCUSSION

As expected, both groups of dysarthric speakers included in this study had significantly longer mean syllable durations than did the normal speakers. These results are consistent with earlier studies which had reported perceptual (Darley et al., 1969), acoustic (Kent & Netsell, 1975;

TABLE 7-2
Mean intelligibility and naturalness ratings for individual subjects in the three groups.

Subject	INTELLIGIBILITY			NATURALNESS		
	Normal	Spastic	Ataxic	Normal	Spastic	Ataxic
1	7.0	6.0	5.2	6.6	4.8	4.4
2	7.0	5.4	5.2	6.8	2.8	2.8
3	7.0	3.6	6.2	7.0	2.2	5.0
4	7.0	2.6	4.4	7.0	1.2	2.6
5	7.0	6.8	4.8	6.8	6.2	3.8
6	6.8	6.2	4.4	6.6	4.6	1.6
7	7.0	6.6	5.0	7.0	5.2	2.8
8	7.0	6.6	5.6	6.8	6.4	4.0
9	7.0	6.4	5.6	6.4	6.0	4.4
10	6.8	4.8	6.0	5.2	2.2	4.4
11	6.8	5.4	5.2	6.6	3.2	3.6
12	7.0	5.6	6.6	6.8	4.4	5.6
13	7.0	4.8	5.8	6.4	2.8	3.8
14	6.8	6.4	6.6	6.4	4.8	5.6
X̄	6.9	5.9	5.7	6.7	4.5	4.2

Kent, Netsell, & Abbs, 1978), and cineradiographic (Kent, et al., 1975) evidence for reduced articulation rate in dysarthria.

The failure to observe a significant difference between the mean syllable durations for the spastic and ataxic dysarthric groups is not in accord with the findings of Darley et al. (1969). These investigators rated the speech of their spastic dysarthric subjects significantly slower than that of their ataxic dysarthric group. Conversely, the findings of the present study are consistent with those of Portnoy and Aronson (1982) who observed no significant difference in mean syllable durations obtained during diadochokinetic tasks between their spastic and ataxic dysarthric subjects.

In considering the discrepancy between the results of Darley et al. (1969) and those of Portnoy and Aronson (1982) and the present study, it is important to note that all three studies had several subjects in common. One possible explanation for the difference in results may lie in the range of severity exhibited by the dysarthric subjects. In the present study, the overall mean intelligibility rating was 5.9 for the spastic and 5.7 for the ataxic dysarthric speakers, with ranges of 2.6-6.8 and 4.4-6.6, respectively. The distribution of subjects across the full range of severity was somewhat uneven, particularly toward the severe end of the continuum. Thus, it may be suggested that inclusion of more severely dysarthric subjects of both types studied would have yielded a greater difference in mean syllable duration. This explanation does not appear to apply to the Portnoy and Aronson study, however. They reported that their subjects had been judged to represent "a reasonably broad range of severity" (p. 325).

A more plausible explanation for the discrepancy between these test results lies in differences among the types of measurement employed. In both the present study and that of Portnoy and Aronson, mean syllable durations were derived from instrumental measurements of the audible portion of the speech sample. The measure of speaking rate employed by Darley et al. (1969) was the perceptual ratings of their subjects' rate of contextual speech. The measures of speaking rate employed were, therefore, not equivalent. In the present study and that of Portnoy and Aronson, rate was determined solely from the audible portions of the speech sample. Darley, Aronson, and Brown's ratings were based on both the audible and inaudible portions of the speech sample. Thus, the significant differences in speech rate between spastic and ataxic dysarthric speakers observed by Darley et al. may have reflected differences in the inaudible portions of the speech sample rather than differences in the audible portions. It may be hypothesized that spastic and ataxic dysarthric speakers, as groups, do not differ in their articulation rates but do differ in the length of their intra- and interword pause times. This is a matter for further investigation.

A second aspect of the results of this study which deserves discussion is the relationship between mean syllable duration and the ratings of intelligibility and naturalness. In this study, mean syllable duration was correlated significantly with both intelligibility and naturalness for the spastic dysarthric speakers. However, neither of these correlations were significant for the ataxic dysarthric group. These results indicate a more consistent relationship between reduced articulation rate and intelligibility and naturalness for the spastic than for the ataxic dysarthric subjects — in spite of almost identical overall mean syllable durations for the two groups. While no direct causal relationship may be inferred from these results, one may speculate that reduced articulation rate contributes more to the diminution of intelligibility and naturalness for spastic dysarthric speakers than it does for ataxic dysarthric speakers. Note, however, that the modest correlations between articulation rate and intelligibility and naturalness leave much room for other, perhaps more important, contributing factors.

This hypothesis has a potentially valuable clinical implication. It may be suggested that various parameters of dysarthric speech may contribute differentially to intelligibility and naturalness in different forms of dysarthria. Perhaps the various aberrant elements of a dysarthric individual's speech combine to form a particular "acoustic-perceptual context" in which certain elements, or combinations of elements, have a more profound effect on intelligibility and naturalness than they would in a different "acoustic-perceptual context." Should this prove to be the case, the efficacy of dysarthria rehabilitation might be enhanced by focusing on those elements of a particular patient's speech that contribute most to decreased intelligibility and naturalness. This suggests the need for additional studies in which the relationships between various parameters of dysarthric speech production and intelligibility and naturalness are assessed.

REFERENCES

Darley, F.L., Aronson, A.E., & Brown, J.R. Differential diagnostic patterns of dysarthria. *Journal of Speech and Hearing Research*, 1969, *12*, 246-269.

Kent, R.D. & Netsell, R. A case study of an ataxic dysarthric: Cineradiographic and spectrographic observations. *Journal of Speech and Hearing Disorders*, 1975, *40*, 115-134.

Kent, R.D., Netsell, R., & Abbs, J. *Acoustic description of segmental and suprasegmental features of ataxic dysarthria.* Paper presented to the annual convention of the American Speech-Language-Hearing Association. San Francisco, 1978.

Kent, R.D., Netsell, R., & Bauer, L.L. Cineradiographic assessment of articulatory mobility in the dysarthrias. *Journal of Speech and Hearing Disorders,* 1975, *40,* 467-480.

Portnoy, R.A. & Aronson, A.E. Diadochokinetic syllable rate and regularity in normal and in spastic and ataxic dysarthric speakers. *Journal of Speech and Hearing Disorders,* 1982, *47,* 324-328.

Siegel, S. *Nonparametric statistics for the behavioral sciences.* New York: McGraw-Hill, 1956.

Winer, B.J. *Statistical principles in experimental design.* New York: McGraw-Hill, 1971.

ACKNOWLEDGMENT

The authors wish to thank Dr. Robert Portnoy for making available the recorded speech samples used in this study. We also extend our thanks to Dr. James Hillis for his assistance in developing the instrumental measurement procedure used in the study and in the statistical analysis of the results.

8

Role of Feedback, Reinforcement, and Compliance on Training and Transfer in Biofeedback-Based Rehabilitation of Motor Speech Disorders

Rick Rubow

INTRODUCTION

Biofeedback is a process of transducing some physiologic variable, transforming the signal to extract useful information, and displaying that information to the subject in a format that will facilitate learning to regulate the physiological variable. Biofeedback techniques, although relatively new, are being used in many fields of medicine and allied health, such as physical therapy, occupational therapy, and psychology. Biofeedback is also being increasingly used in the treatment of speech disorders. Its use is limited, however, by sparse literature on treatment efficacy as well as poor understanding of the biofeedback process. There is a need to explore when, how (and if) it can be used effectively.

In speech rehabilitation, we commonly ask patients to voluntarily control a specific component of the speech system. Unfortunately, little is known regarding the normal voluntary control of these components. One purpose of the present study was to collect empirical data on normal subjects as a benchmark for evaluating dysfunction in dysarthrics.

Much of the emphasis in previous biofeedback studies has been based on what the subject learns; less attention has been given to *how* the subject learns. As treatment methods do not exist in a vacuum, but follow from a conceptual framework, determining an appropriate model of the biofeedback process would optimize its use as a treatment technique. Thus, the second purpose of this study was to test some of the underlying assumptions of several biofeedback models as they might apply to the treatment of motor-speech disorders.

A number of models have been advanced to explain biofeedback processes, such as cognitive mediation, somatic mediation, operant conditioning, and servocontrol. Each one focuses on somewhat different areas, but vague semantic distinctions inevitably blur the boundaries between them. It is beyond the scope of this chapter to describe these models and the literature supporting them in detail, but a brief account of two models is necessary to provide a perspective from which to view the specific research questions to be considered.

Operant Conditioning versus Cybernetic Model

Operant conditioning and cybernetic models represent fundamentally different approaches to conceptualizing the biofeedback process. The operant conditioning model simply extends to biofeedback the concepts of reinforcement and temporal contiguity underlying classical and operant conditioning (Black, Cott, & Pavloski, 1977). Cybernetic models, on the other hand, conceptualize biofeedback in terms of continuous closed-loop processes. The motor skills model (Lang, 1974) and the hierarchical control models (Schwartz, 1976; Smith & Henry, 1967; Tatten & Lee, 1975) are examples of this latter type. It should be noted that cybernetic models as applied to biofeedback are more concerned with the acquisition of new behavior than with the execution of well-established behaviors. Even though some rapid motor sequences normally may be executed open-loop, such behavior may have been acquired under closed-loop control. Similarly, the rehabilitation of movement patterns that normally could be executed open-loop involves the relearning of new, perhaps compensatory, patterns under closed-loop control.

Past research. One goal of this study was to determine which of the two model types — operant conditioning or cybernetic — is more appropriate in explaining biofeedback processes. A critical issue in distinguishing between these model types is the relative importance a model assigns to reinforcement and dynamic feedback. Biofeedback literature supports the roles of both reinforcement and information feedback, but most of this support stems from the *terminology* chosen by various authors to reflect their theoretical approach rather than from experimental evidence. Still, a few studies have shed light on the issue. For example, Kondo, Travis, and Knott (1975) provided subjects with auditory feedback of alpha brainwave activity and rewarded increases in alpha with different amounts of money. Alpha production increased in all groups, but the amount of the reward had no differential effect on the amount of alpha production. Other studies reported similar results for alpha training (Regestein, Pegram, Cook, & Bradley, 1973) and EMG training (Malec, Sipprelle, & Behring, 1978). Although these studies experimentally manipulated reinforcement conditions, they confounded the roles of reinforcement and feedback. The critical experiments needed to separate these constructs have not yet been conducted. Separating these constructs is not trivial, as the biofeedback signal contains information about performance that may also serve to reinforce behavior change in the direction of a target behavior.

A study by Rubow and Smith (1971), however, did separate the effects of reinforcement and feedback — not by varying the amount of reinforcement, but by manipulating the temporal and informational characteristics of the biofeedback display. For an operant conditioning model, reinforcement is effective if it is provided within a few seconds of a desired response. For cybernetic models, continuous and immediate information about performance is the key to perceptual-motor learning. The Rubow and Smith study compared subjects' ability to control electromyographic signals under two conditions of visual feedback. A moving average display provided continuous feedback of EMG (delayed by the averaging process). An intermittent average display summarized a similar quantity of information, but introduced discrete delays between updates of the display. Since the delays were less than 750 msec for both displays, indicating that their reinforcing properties are similar, an operant conditioning model predicts no performance differences between them. A cybernetic model, on the other hand, predicts improved performance for the continuous display. The results of Rubow and Smith (1971) indicated superior performance for continuous feedback, but transfer of training to a no-feedback condition was not measured.

Current study. The present study also assessed the role of feedback and reinforcement by manipulating the temporal and informational characteristics of a feedback display. Both training and transfer of training to a no-feedback condition were measured. More specifically, learning and retention were compared under conditions of continuous visual feedback of performance and under visual knowledge of results of performance. In this paradigm, the amount and nature of the information displayed to the subject was equivalent in both conditions. The crucial difference was the temporal relationship between performance (motor output) and information about that output. Subjects in the visual feedback condition received continuous information within one msec of output. In contrast, subjects in the knowledge of results condition received the identical display of output over the course of the five-sec. trial, except that they saw a static trace of their performance only after the motor output had been completed. The average time lag was 2.5 sec. Thus, differences in learning between visual feedback and knowledge of results (KR) groups could not be attributed to sensory modality, or to the amount of information contained in the display. An operant conditioning model predicts no differences between conditions, because the requirements of temporal contiguity necessary for reinforcement and learning are equally satisfied under both conditions. A cybernetic model predicts superior performance under the condition of continuous dynamic feedback because, in such models, this type of information is continuously integrated into the subjects' ongoing motor control processes.

In order to answer the question of feedback vs. reinforcement as it relates to speech, it was necessary to define a relevant training task. As stated earlier, when biofeedback is used to treat a motor-speech disorder, patients are asked to improve control of some component of the speech system (e.g., Netsell & Daniel, 1979). Respiration was chosen for this study, because respiratory control is a prerequisite for most other interventions. Training in respiratory control, rather than in a speaking task, also eliminated the possible confounding of intrinsic acoustic with extrinsic visual feedback.

Based on the limited literature supporting the role of continuous feedback in learning and the negative results of studies that manipulated the amount of reinforcement, it was expected that continuous dynamic feedback would result in superior learning and transfer of training as compared with static knowledge of results.

Compliant versus Noncompliant Feedback

One goal of this study was to test certain assumptions of operant conditioning and cybernetic models of biofeedback. A second goal was to test additional tenets of a cybernetic model. More specifically, this study tested the robustness of the compliance principle of motor skills learning (see Smith & Smith, 1973). The sensorimotor compliance principle, as applied to biofeedback, states that learning is more efficient when the augmented sensory consequences of motor output (biofeedback) are compliant with (or similar to) the sensory consequences normally accompanying that motor output. That is, compliant biofeedback could be more easily integrated with the intrinsic feedback normally generated by the human control system. An example of noncompliant feedback would be an increase in the loudness of a buzzer to indicate increased muscle relaxation to the subject. The arousing feedback here is not compliant with the goal of relaxation. In contrast, the commonly used compliant feedback indicator of muscle relaxation is an auditory signal that decreases in pitch proportionately with increased relaxation. In this case, the soothing lower-pitched tones serve to enhance relaxation behavior and thus are compliant with the training goal.

In order to increase the efficiency of data collection, the compliance principle was tested with the same training task used in the feedback versus reinforcement part of the study. Since the hypothesis posed was that visual feedback is superior to visual KR, the compliance hypothesis was tested by comparing two types of feedback displays.

In a training task involving control of respiration, the compliance principle predicts that auditory feedback will be superior to visual feedback because the intrinsic sensory consequences of respiration are primarily auditory rather than visual. The compliance principle further predicts that intensity, rather than frequence coding, of that auditory feedback will be superior because increased expiratory effort results in increased intensity of intrinsic respiratory sounds, as well as increased intensity of speech.

This aspect of the study compared the performance of subjects receiving visual feedback of expiration rate with that of subjects receiving auditory intensity feedback. It was expected that, as auditory feedback is more compliant for a respiratory task, it would result in superior learning and transfer of training compared to visual feedback. It should be noted that a comparison of these two displays confounds the amount of information (resolution of error) with sensory modality. The just noticeable difference (JND) is smaller for the visual display than for the auditory display. The aim of this study, however, was not to compare an artificially degraded visual display with an intrinsically lower resolution auditory display. While it was necessary to equate information across displays within the visual modality to answer the feedback versus reinforcement question, such equalization in this case could bias the results in favor of the auditory display, thus indicating a compliance effect not normally present. By contrast, a compliance effect robust enough to compensate for information differences could be clinically useful.

Hypotheses

(1.) In part one of this study, normal subjects were trained to improve respiratory control by means of either a visual feedback display or a visual knowledge of results display. Both displays contained equivalent reinforcing properties, but the feedback display provided continuous information about performance. The hypothesis was that feedback would result in superior performance when compared to knowledge of results. This finding would support a cybernetic model based on feedback rather than an operant conditioning model based on reinforcement as the more appropriate way to conceptualize biofeedback.

(2.) The second part of this study tested the cybernetic principle of compliance. A group of normal subjects was trained to improve respiratory control by means of either a visual or auditory display. The auditory display was considered to be more compliant with respiratory control than the visual display, because the normal sensory consequences of respiration are auditory rather than visual. Therefore, the hypothesis was that auditory feedback would result in superior respiratory control compared to visual.

METHOD

Experimental Design

The experimental paradigm used to assess learning and transfer of training for the different training conditions involved measuring pretraining performance on a motor control task, providing training with different displays, and measuring posttraining performance. There are many ways to operationally define transfer. As is often the case in scientific experiments, the same data can generate different conclusions, depending on the specific definitions used (Andreas, 1960). One paradigm involves practicing on the training condition until specific criteria are met on the transfer task. The number of training trials to meet criteria is the measure of transfer. Another paradigm ranks the absolute value of the final performance scores for each group. One problem with this method is that it does not take into account pretraining differences. To overcome this problem, the change between pre- and posttraining scores can be compared. This method is subject to ceiling effects. One problem with all methods that use the absolute value of the performance scores is that it is impossible to compare data across studies. Thus, transforming absolute scores into percentages provides more useful data.

The definition of transfer used in this study required a control group trained for an equivalent amount of time on the posttest task. The dependent variable, percentage Direct Practice Increment, is the difference between the control group pretest and the experimental group posttest, divided by the difference between the control group pre- and posttest (Andreas, 1960). This percentage DPI can be expressed as follows: $\%DPI = (C_i\text{-}E) / (C_i\text{-}C_e)$ where C_i = initial performance on pretest for the control group, C_e = posttest for the control group, and E = posttest for the experimental group. It should be noted that the control group does not necessarily provide a comparison between feedback and no-feedback, but allows one to subtract the effects of variables common to all groups from the independent variables of training display.

The posttest was delayed for 10 minutes, and results were compared with performance on the same task at the end of training (EOT). This provided a measure of shortterm transfer for each group. Three types of training modes (visual, auditory, knowledge of results), each with a different form of display, were compared.

Tracking Paradigms

Besides defining transfer operationally, it was also necessary to define a specific training task. A *tracking paradigm* is a convenient way to do this. The three basic elements of any tracking paradigm are: target, cursor, and error detector. The target represents a predefined motor output required of the subject. It can take the form of movement in a particular spatial pattern, or it can represent a pattern of change of any physiologic variable that is under the subject's voluntary control. The cursor represents the subject's motor or physiologic output as measured by a transducer. The error detector represents a comparison of the target with the cursor when both are represented in similar physical units (e.g., voltage). There are two types of tracking paradigms, each differing in the way error information is displayed to the subject. In *pursuit tracking*, the target and cursor are displayed as distinctly different signals so the subject can experience his or her effort to control the cursor without confounding it with the target. The subject compares the two signals to calculate error. In *compensatory tracking*, the error signal, or difference between target and cursor, is calculated by the display device and displayed as one signal. Thus, the subject experiences only the direction and magnitude of error, but not the required target.

It is not clear which type of tracking paradigm is most compatible with speech production. Models of speech production differ greatly in their assumptions. For example, MacNeilage (1970) proposed a primarily open-loop model in which speech was coded as spatial targets. Other models defined speech in terms of acoustic or perceptual targets (Lindblom, 1963; Nooteboom, 1970/1980) or in terms of afference referenced to motor commands (Fairbanks, 1954). In all these models the control system compared some form of target with some form of cursor. Therefore, a pursuit, rather than a compensatory tracking paradigm, seemed more appropriate for speech motor control and was used in the present study.

Tracking Error

In both pursuit and compensatory tracking, performance is measured by comparing the target and cursor values at selected moments in time and by averaging these momentary errors over longer spans of time. In a computerized paradigm, time is divided into discrete units as defined by a real-time sampling clock. At each "tick" of the clock, the computer samples the target and cursor values and computes the difference between them. If the cursor is leading the target, the sign if positive; if it is lagging the target, the sign is negative. These values form the primary data for summary over longer time intervals. A simple method of analysis is to add the values algebraically. One problem with this approach is that the net error over time sums to zero if the net positive error and net negative error are equal. One way to overcome this problem is to sum the absolute value of the error. Another method is to calculate the root mean square or RMS error. In this approach, each momentary error value is squared or multiplied by itself (converting negative to positive values) and then summed over a time interval. The square root of the sum is the final error. This method weights extreme error scores more than small error scores in the summing process, thus magnifying learning effects. More complex analysis of error data can extract gain and phase differences between the target and cursor, thus separating correct but delayed responses from incorrect responses. Since constant value targets were used in this study such complex analysis was not warranted, and the sum of absolute error was used. More specifically, absolute error was averaged over 1-second intervals, and the first interval of each trial was not scored.

Subjects

From a pool of volunteers, 24 subjects ranging from 21 to 35 years of age were selected who could pass an audiometric screening test (hearing loss less than 5 dBHL bilaterally at .5, 1, 2, 4, and 8 KHz and 0 dBHL at 250Hz). These subjects were then randomly assigned to one of three training groups or to a control group. No attempt was made to control for sex or age. All subjects were naive as to the nature and purpose of the study and had no prior biofeedback experience. Two cerebral palsied-dysarthric subjects were also trained on the respiratory control task. Both subjects were ambulatory, in their mid-40's, of above average intelligence, and had moderate limb involvement and dysarthria. One subject was predominantly spastic and the other had both spastic and athetoid involvement.

Equipment

The subject's task was to exhale for 5 sec at specified rates through a leak tube 5 cm long and 2 mm internal diameter. Intra-oral air pressure (P_o), measured with a Statham PM 131 transducer, was used as the measure of expiration rate, as described by Netsell and Hixon (1978). This pressure information was provided for the subjects via different displays, depending on their assigned training group.

A storage oscilloscope (Tektronix T912) provided the visual feedback. Upward vertical movement of a light spot indicated increased P_o, and downward movement indicated decreased P_o. A second light spot indicated the target respiration. The gain was adjusted so that one cm of water pressure equaled .8 cm of vertical displacement on the scope screen. Both spots also moved from left to right across the 10 cm screen at the rate of 2 cm per sec so that the entire 5-sec trial could be displayed on one sweep with maximum resolution. The scope was set to memory mode, so in addition to the immediate feedback, persisting traces of respiration and target remained on the screen until the end of the trial. The subject viewed an image of the oscilloscope screen via closed-circuit TV.

The knowledge of results (KR) display was identical to the visual display with one exception: the subjects did not view the display until immediately after the end of each trial. Thus, they did not receive real-time biofeedback, but only static knowledge of results of their past, completed performance.

Auditory feedback consisted of a 250Hz sine wave presented binaurally through Koss Pro-4A headphones. The target was represented in the left ear by a constant intensity tone, and the subject's pressure was represented in the right ear as a variable intensity tone with increased intensity proportional to increased pressure. The targets ranged in intensity from 55 to 65 dBSPL.

A real-time computer system was used to automate the training paradigm. It generated the different targets, indicated the beginning and end of trials and rest periods, controlled the training displays, and summarized the subject's performance data for further analysis. The computer (PDP 8) was interfaced with the electronic equipment by means of digital relays and analog-digital and digital-analog converters.

The software used was custom designed to implement tracking paradigms. A major feature is flexibility: elements of the paradigm may be varied without having to rewrite segments of code. This flexibility was achieved by designing a series of "virtual devices" that can be linked together in different ways via a programming control language designed for tracking studies.

Procedure

The experimental session for each subject consisted of six sets of trials. First, the details of the pressure-matching task were explained. The subjects were instructed to breathe as they normally would in a resting state. Their task was learning to inhale to the same depth prior to the start of a trial, and then to exhale through a mouthpiece/leak tube configuration at a specified constant rate for the 5-sec duration of the trial. Three different rates or targets within the range experienced during normal speaking were defined. The target values corresponded to expiration rates of 66, 100, and 133 cc per second. The subjects were told that, although they would receive information about their respiration during training, their ultimate goal was to learn to reproduce the three targets without external feedback.

Next, the subjects were familiarized with the computer-generated instructions for each trial. The computer generated a 2-sec warble tone through headphones to the left ear. This indicated that a trial was about to begin and that the subject should begin inspiration. After 2-secs, the computer generated a second warble tone, and the trial began when the second tone ended. Five seconds later, the end of the trial was signaled by a warble tone. During the trial, the information displayed to the subject varied, depending on the condition and group. During all trials, a red LED was turned on to give additional indication that the subject was supposed to be performing the respiration task. This extra cue was particularly important during the no-feedback trials.

After this explanation, subjects underwent five practice trials with the computer to insure that they understood the task. To prevent this familiarization process from contaminating the pretest performance, a manual task was used. Subjects were required not to generate the target via respiration, but to move a control lever in the vertical dimension with thumb and forefinger. The training display for each group was similar to the experimental display.

After becoming familiar with the basic elements of the task, but before they had practiced the respiratory task, the subjects were given a pretest on the respiratory task. This test consisted of one trial containing all three display conditions (visual, auditory, and KR), followed by five trials of no feedback or KR. This sequence was repeated for each target level, for a total of 18 trials. The displays were presented on trials 1, 7, and 12 to enable the subject to find the "ballpark" approximation to the correct target. The training consisted of refining the initial estimates of correct respiratory effort. Performance on the 15 no-feedback trials constituted the pretest scores.

The training phase of the study consisted of three sets of 18 trials (one set for each target). The sequence within the set was five trials of the display condition assigned to the group (visual, auditory, KR, or control), followed by one trial of KR. This six-trial sequence was repeated three times per set. The single KR trial was necessary to keep the control group in the "ballpark," and was also incorporated into the experimental groups to maintain equivalence of training.

After completing the three training sets, all groups rested for 10 minutes and then received the posttest. This consisted of one trial of visual and auditory feedback, plus KR followed by five trials of no feedback or KR. The sequence was repeated for each target. The posttest was identical to the pretest.

RESULTS

Normal Data

One of the more striking results was the large variability in performance across subjects. Figure 8-1 shows five trials of pretest and five trials of posttest performance for one of the more proficient subjects. Some less proficient subjects were out of range of the oscilloscope for some trials.

Four subjects (one from each group) were eliminated from the analysis based on extreme pretest error scores compared to the mean for all subjects. These individuals were unable to perform the relatively simple respiratory control task and often generated maximum possible error scores of 2,000 units. Their error scores ranged from greater than 1.5 to 3 standard deviations above the group mean. The remaining subjects were within one standard deviation. The mean and standard deviation of error within group are summarized in Table 8-1. Although some learning did occur, as evidenced by the decrease in both mean and variance from pretest to posttest scores, even the best performance was variable. A constant error of 1 cm water pressure equals 256 error units.

The percentage DPI was calculated for each group relative to the control group as discussed in the **Method** section. The results shown in Figure 8-2 indicate that visual feedback was superior to KR. The difference between conditions was tested using the Two Sample t Test (Ryan, Joiner, & Ryan, 1976). Unlike the standard t Test, this test does not require homogeneity of variance. The difference in transfer of training between visual feedback and KR conditions was significant at $p > .05$. The difference between auditory and visual feedback was significant at $p > .05$.

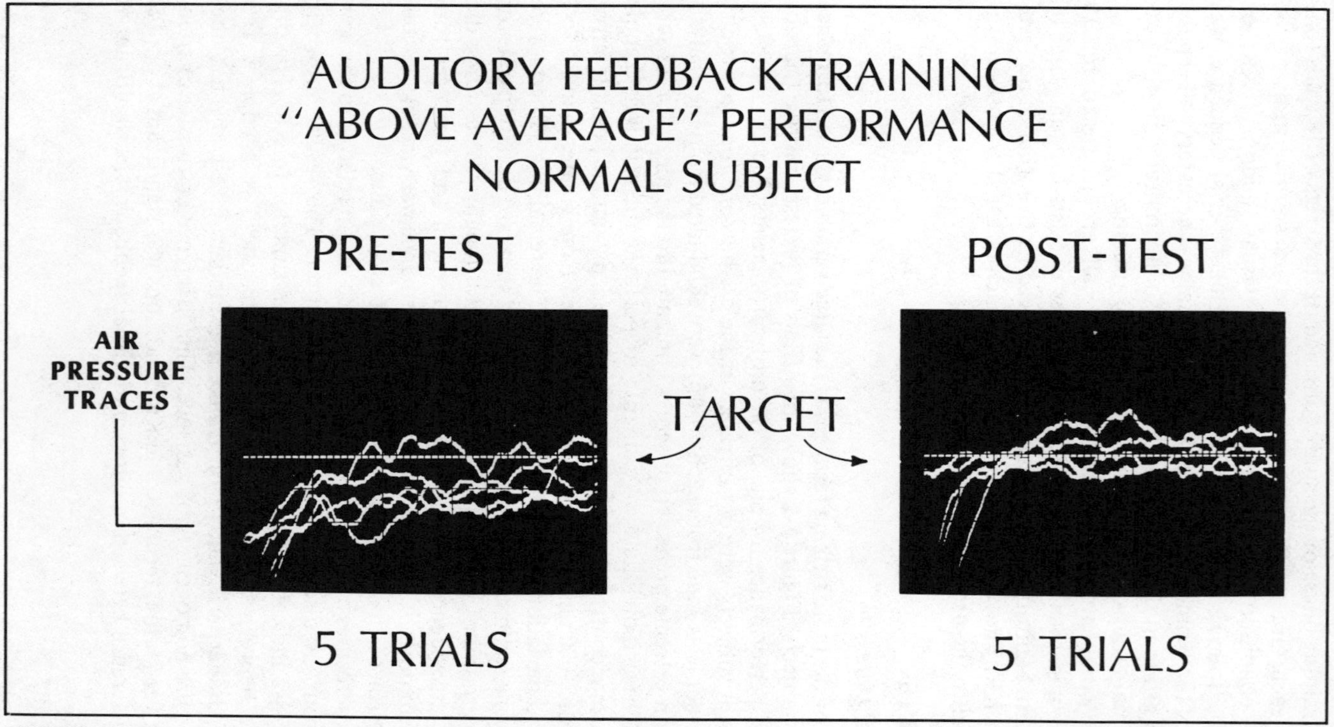

AUDITORY FEEDBACK TRAINING
"ABOVE AVERAGE" PERFORMANCE
NORMAL SUBJECT

PRE-TEST

POST-TEST

5 TRIALS

5 TRIALS

TARGET

AIR PRESSURE TRACES

FIGURE 8-1
Oscilloscope traces of expiration during the no-feedback trials before and after training for an above average normal subject.

TABLE 8-1
Means and standard deviations of tracking error before and after training and at the delayed posttest, averaged for each display condition.

GROUP	PRETEST	EOT	POSTTEST
KR	315,SD = 111	158,SD = 100	330,SD = 181
VISUAL	383,SD = 271	287,SD = 247	247,SD = 100
AUDITORY	399,SD = 231	182,SD = 107	289,SD = 132

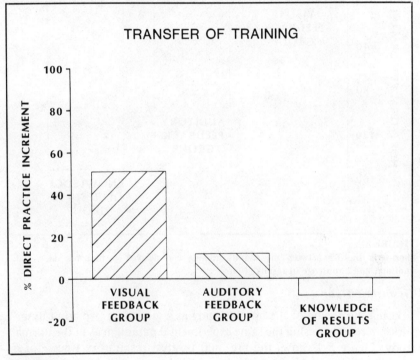

FIGURE 8-2
Percentage Direct Practice Increment for the visual, auditory and knowledge of results groups.

Short-term transfer is defined as the difference between the no-feedback performance immediately at the end of the training (EOT) and the posttest administered 10 minutes after the end of training. Figure 8-3 shows that the visual group retained their performance while the KR and auditory groups did not. The performance decrement for both groups was significant at $p > .05$.

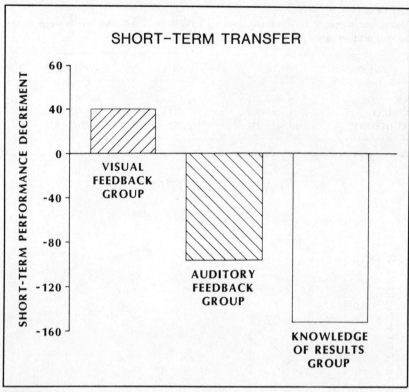

FIGURE 8-3
Short-term transfer between the end of training and delayed posttest for the visual, auditory, and knowledge of results groups.

Dysarthric Data

Using the results of the normal study as a guideline, two adult dysarthrics were tested using the same experimental paradigm as in the normal study. Figure 8-4 shows the pre- and posttest respiratory traces for a cerebral palsied adult with both athetoid and spastic involvement (mixed) who had been trained on visual feedback. Learning was characterized by a relative decrease in variability although there was no improvement in absolute accuracy. Figure 8-5 shows pre- and posttest traces for a predominantly athetoid cerebral palsied adult who had also been trained on visual feedback.

The transfer of training data for the dysarthric subjects is displayed in a different format than the normal data. Since the control group was not comparable, the percentage DPI measure could not be calculated for the dysarthrics. One major difference was that their respiratory control was

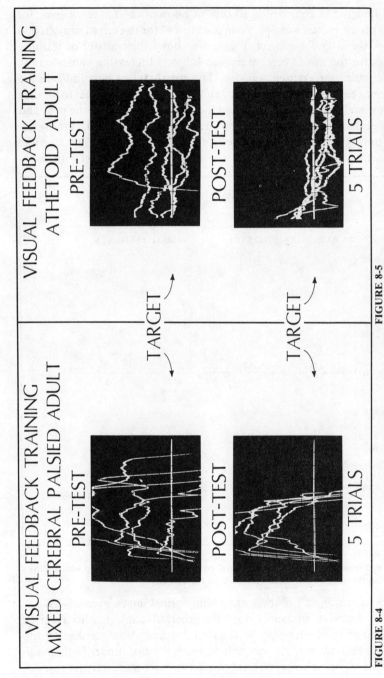

VISUAL FEEDBACK TRAINING
ATHETOID ADULT

PRE-TEST

POST-TEST

5 TRIALS

TARGET

TARGET

VISUAL FEEDBACK TRAINING
MIXED CEREBRAL PALSIED ADULT

PRE-TEST

POST-TEST

5 TRIALS

FIGURE 8-4
Oscilloscope traces of expiration during the no-feedback trials before and after visual feedback training for a cerebral palsied adult with athetoid and spastic involvement (mixed).

FIGURE 8-5
Oscilloscope traces of expiration during no-feedback trials before and after visual feedback training for an athetoid cerebral palsied adult.

greatly impaired in comparison to that of normals. The average error for normals on the pretest was 366, compared to 740 for the mixed subject, and 1,020 for the athetoid subject. Figure 8-6 shows the transfer of training measures for the mixed cerebal palsied subject. Increasing values on the ordinate indicate increased transfer. The crosshatched bars indicate the difference between the pre-test and end-of-training performance measures, and the open bars indicate the difference between the pre- and posttest performance measures. The figure illustrates that no learning occurred during the first training session with auditory feedback, while some learning occurred during the second day training session with visual

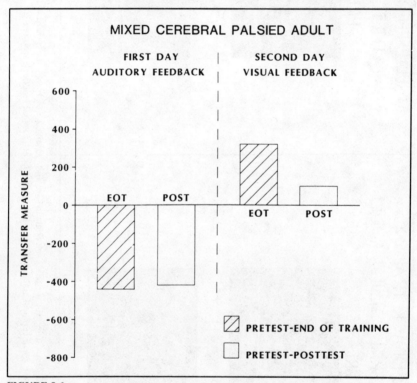

FIGURE 8-6
Training and transfer measures for the mixed cerebral palsied adult trained with auditory feedback on the 1st day and visual feedback on the 2nd day.

feedback. The subject's hearing was within normal limits. Figure 8-7 shows the same transfer measures for the athetoid subject who received knowledge of results training on the first day and visual feedback training on the second day. He was able to learn the task under both conditions. This subject, however, experienced a short-term transfer loss for the visual condition rather than for the knowledge of results condition, in contrast with the normal data.

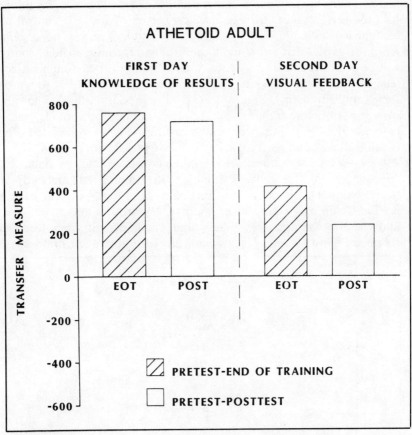

FIGURE 8-7
Training and transfer measures for the athetoid cerebral palsied adult trained with knowledge of results on the 1st day and visual feedback on the 2nd day.

DISCUSSION

The results of this study indicated that for a respiratory control task, visual feedback training resulted in superior transfer to a no-feedback condition as compared to visual knowledge of results and auditory feedback training. On one level, these results represent an empirical comparison of specific training techniques applicable to respiration. The data also provide an empirical measure of how well normal subjects can control expiratory air flow. It is important to distinguish measures of unaided regulation from measures obtained with the aid of external information such as feedback or knowledge of results. This distinction is particularly important if one wishes to make comparisons or inferences between normal and abnormal function. If comparisons are made under visual feedback of performance, for example, properties of intrinsic control are confounded with those of visual-motor control. There is no *a priori* reason to expect that visual-motor control and intrinsic unaided control will be similarly impaired in abnormals. Pearson product-moment correlation coefficients for visual feedback and no-feedback trials within the same set illustrate this point (at least for linear relationships). The value of r was .49 before training and .11 after training for normals, and .7 before and after training for the dysarthrics. The correspondence between feedback and no-feedback conditions varied with performance.

We must also be cautious about relating normals' ability or inability to improve control with feedback training to the training potential of dysarthrics. Normal subjects may be functioning at or near physiological upper limits and may be unable to improve. Dysarthrics may function via idiosyncratic compensatory modes and might benefit from feedback training. Figure 8-8 shows the tracking error for both dysarthric subjects

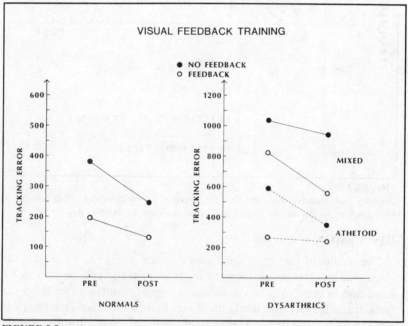

FIGURE 8-8
Absolute tracking error before and after visual feedback training for the group of normals and the dysarthric subjects. The feedback and no-feedback conditions were within the same set of trials. Note the reduced scale for the dysarthric subjects.

and the normal group trained with visual feedback. Note the reduced scale for the dysarthrics. The figure shows that although the final performance of the athetoid subject was no better than the pretraining level of normals, his absolute improvement was greater. The figure also illustrates the problems in predicting training potential from performance with feedback. The athetoid subject made little improvement on the feedback condition, but improved considerably on the no-feedback post-test. By contrast, the mixed subject improved with feedback but had relatively little carry-over to no-feedback.

Perhaps the most interesting feature of the data is the large variability, even across normal subjects. This variability is consistent with results of other studies designed to assess the role of intrinsic feedback in speech production (e.g., Garber, Speidel, Siegel, Miller, & Glass, 1980). Although statistically significant differences between groups were found in the present study, there may be strong, idiosyncratic differences in an individual's ability to process various forms of sensory information. If these differences override general principles of rehabilitation techniques, it may be necessary to empirically match specific biofeedback displays to individual patients in order to optimize training.

Compliant versus Noncompliant Feedback

More generally, this study tested certain assumptions of different models of biofeedback. One assumption tested was the sensorimotor compliance principle as applied to respiratory control. This principle states that auditory intensity feedback is superior to visual feedback, because the normal sensory consequences of respiration are auditory rather than visual.

The results showed that differences in performance between visual and auditory feedback training were statistically significant. The trend, although characterized by a high degree of variability, indicated visual feedback as superior to auditory. Clearly, the sensorimotor compliance hypothesis was not supported. It may be that the greater amount of feedback information available in the visual display was more important for learning. These results, coupled with the observations of other investigators that auditory feedback given during speaking tasks may interfere with the processing of normal acoustic information (e.g., Prosek, Montgomery, Walden, & Schwartz, 1978) suggest a diminished role for auditory biofeedback in speech rehabilitation. Other forms of the compliance principle, however, are yet to be explored.

Operant Conditioning versus Cybernetic Model

The biofeedback signal incorporates two constructs related to learning—information about performance and reinforcement for good performance. The specific role of these constructs has not been clearly distinguished in the literature. Often the terms *feedback* (central to cybernetic models) and *reinforcement* (central to an operant conditioning model) are used synonymously. Since distinguishing between these concepts may be critical to the effective planning of treatment, it may be useful to review their definitions.

Reinforcement is defined as "something" that increases the probability that a given response will occur. Thorndike's "Law of Effect" (1898/1973) forms the empirical basis of reinforcement. Simply stated, this principle asserts that events followed by satisfying consequences are likely to be repeated. Temporal contiguity, a second feature of reinforcement, refers to the requirement that a reinforcer must occur within a relatively short time period after a response is emitted in order for learning to occur. Learning is defined as a change in the probability that the response will occur.

A major conceptual difficulty with reinforcement is its tautological nature. Reinforcement can only be defined as "something" which increases the probability of a response. Whether a specific "something" qualifies as a reinforcer cannot be determined as an independent property, but only empirically for each situation. For example, the studies described in the Introduction, showing no differential effect of amount of monetary reward on EMG and alpha control can simply be interpreted as empirical evidence that the money was not a reinforcer for those subjects. Thus, the reinforcement concept is very robust because it is difficult to experimentally reject. It is limited in usefulness, however, because of its inability to predict conditions for optimum learning.

The concept of feedback is distinctly different from reinforcement. These differences were summarized by K. U. Smith (e.g., Smith & Henry, 1967), whose theoretical framework and computerized research techniques predated the development of biofeedback.[1] Smith defined three types of feedback—reactive, operational, and instrumental. The afferent signals generated by an individual's own bodily movements and unaided behavior are referred to as reactive feedback. When the individual is using a tool, the feedback received from the action of that tool is referred to as instrumental. The persisting effect of a tool—using operation on objects or materials in the environment is operational feedback. Reactive and instrumental feedback are dynamic changing patterns generated by the moving parts of the body and the moving tool. Operational feedback arises from the results of the behavior and thus persists as a static pattern after the dynamic motion that produced it has ceased. Instrumental feedback corresponds to the concept of biofeedback and operational feedback corresponds to the concept of reinforcement.

One major difference between dynamic feedback and reinforcement is the precision of the temporal requirements for learning. While reinforcement is effective if provided within seconds (or even minutes) after a response, feedback delays of fractions of a second can impair performance. Intermittency effects are also different. Intermittent reinforcement increases the stability of a response and decreases extinction rate. By contrast, intermittent external feedback does not produce this effect.

Another difference stems from the tautological nature of reinforcement. Reinforcement can be defined and measured only in terms of its demonstrated effects on learning in particular situations. By contrast, the closed-loop factors, determinants of learning in cybernetic models, can be qualitatively and quantitatively described in terms of measurable variations in spatial, temporal, and kinetic feedback patterns.

The results of this study indicate that continuous dynamic feedback is superior to static knowledge of results in the learning and short-term retention of a respiratory control task. Because the reinforcement properties of the two displays are similar, the improved performance under the dynamic feedback condition supports a cybernetic rather than an operant conditioning model of the biofeedback process. As indicated above, there are a number of differences between these models that suggest different treatment methods.

An operant conditioning model leads to treatments based on providing extrinsic reinforcers for desired behaviors. Therapists must empirically determine the specific environmental events that are positively reinforcing for each individual—as the model has no provisions for determining reinforcers on an *a priori* basis. The desired behaviors are subdivided into small, discrete steps, and each step in the chain is reinforced. The motivation to perform is assumed to arise from the presence of these external environmental events. Most of the treatments involve three components: attention, imitation, and reinforcement. First, one must insure that the patient is attending to the therapist's behavior. Visual and auditory sensory modalities are most often emphasized (through verbalizations of the therapist). Second, the therapist performs the desired behavior. The therapist is limited to a small portion of the relevant behavior associated with speech production and must often exaggerate the components of the behavior in order for the patient to discriminate essential features. Finally, if the task was correctly imitated, the therapist reinforces the patient with verbal praise or some external token. One major problem at this stage is that it is difficult for the therapist to reliably identify small changes in performance and it is difficult to maintain a consistent set of standards for reinforcement. In spite of these problems, the techniques based on an operant conditioning model do work. Other treatments based on a cybernetic model, however, should be explored, especially in difficult cases, for this may lead to more effective methods.

Cybernetic models generate treatment philosophies different from those of the operant conditioning approach. In a cybernetic model, behavior is assumed to be feedback controlled. Speech production is viewed in a similar manner as a multidimensional sensorimotor control process in which both verbal and nonverbal components are integrated to extend control over the environment.

The cybernetic view is that speech production involves feedback relationships with basic body movements and nonverbal activities. Therefore, the fundamental starting point in communication rehabilitation is the *re-establishing of motor control of sensory input in a systematic way.* More specifically, one must provide feedback control loops between the patient and his or her environment that delineate and enhance the patient's self-regulation abilities. In this framework, one can measure motor output from different levels of the speech system and provide dynamic biofeedback via different sensory modalities. Two features of this approach are not considered under operant conditioning. First, close attention must be paid to the critical temporal relationship between motor output and sensory consequences of that output. For example, a Language Master device may provide reinforcement but does not provide dynamic feedback. The reinforcing properties may serve to increase the probability of occurrence of a response, already within the patient's behavioral repertoire, but dynamic sensory feedback is necessary to enable the patient to perform a new behavior. Feedback is more important in early stages of rehabilitation, while the role of reinforcement increases in later stages. A second distinctive feature of the cybernetic approach concerns the repetition of specific movement patterns. While operant conditioning can shape or gradually modify a response already spontaneously emitted by the patient, a cybernetic approach provides the patient with precise information to enable him or her to repeat the identical response many times until it is well established.

These distinctions are particularly important in the treatment of neurogenic speech disorders in which normal neural pathways involved in controlling speech are damaged. Reinforcement does not teach a rat how to press a lever, but only to do so more often. If the feedback information is not available to the control system, no amount of reinforcement can change the behavior. Thus, biofeedback is not just another form of reinforcement, but must be considered as a distinctly different phenomenon. Understanding this difference may be important in optimizing treatment programs.

NOTE

¹The literature supporting these views is referenced in that article and will not be cited here.

REFERENCES

Andreas, B. G. *Experimental psychology.* New York: Wiley & Sons, 1960.

Black, A. M., Cott, A., & Pavloski, R. The operant learning theory approach to biofeedback training. In G. E. Schwartz & J. Beatty (Eds.), *Biofeedback: Theory and research.* New York: Academic Press, 1977, 89-127.

Fairbanks, G. A theory of the speech mechanism as a servosystem. *Journal of Speech and Hearing Disorders,* 1954, *19,* 133-139.

Garber, S. R., Speidel, T. M., Siegel, G. M., Miller, E., & Glass, L. The effects of presentation of noise and dental appliances on speech. *Journal of Speech and Hearing Research,* 1980, *23,* 838-852.

Kondo, C. Y., Travis, T. A., & Knott, J. R. The effect of changes in motivation in alpha enhancement. *Psychophysiology,* 1975, *12,* 388-389.

Lang, P. J. Learned control of human heart rate in a computer directed environment. In P. A. Obrist, A. H. Black, J. Brener, & L. V. DiCara (Eds.), *Cardiovascular psychophysiology.*Chicago: Aldine, 1974, 392-405.

Lindblom, B. E. F. Spectrographic study of vowel reduction. *Journal of the Acoustical Society of America,* 1963, *35,* 1773-1781.

MacNeilage, P. F. Motor control of serial ordering of speech. *Psychological Review,* 1970, *77,* 182-196.

Malec, J., Sipprelle, C. N., & Behring, S. Biofeedback-assisted EMG reduction and subsequent self-disclosure. *Journal of Clinical Psychology,* 1978, *34,* 523-525.

Netsell, R., & Daniel, B. Dysarthria in adults: Physiologic approach to rehabilitation. *Archives of Physical Medicine and Rehabilitation,* 1979, *60,* 500-508.

Netsell, R., & Hixon, T. J. A noninvasive method for clinically estimating subglottal air pressure. *Journal of Speech and Hearing Disorders,* 1978, 326-330.

Nooteboom, S. G. The target theory of speech production. *IPO Annual Progress Report* (Vol. 5). Eindhoven, Netherlands: Institute for Perception Research, 1970, 51-55. (In G. J. Borden & K. S. Harris *Speech science primer.* Baltimore, Maryland: Williams & Wilkins, 1980.)

Prosek, R., Montgomery, A., Walden, B., & Schwartz, D. EMG biofeedback in the treatment of hyperfunctional voice disorders. *Journal of Speech and Hearing Disorders,* 1978, *43,* 282-294.

Regestein, Q. R., Pegram, V., Cook, B., & Bradley, D. Alpha rhythm percentage maintained during 4- and 12-hour feedback periods. *Psychosomatic Medicine,* 1973, *35,* 215-222.

Rubow, R. T., & Smith, K. U. Feedback parameters of electromyographic learning. *American Journal of Physical Medicine,* 1971, *50,* 115-131.

Ryan, T. A., Joiner, B. L., & Ryan, B. F. *Minitab student handbook.* North Seituate, Massachusetts: Duxbury Press, 1976.

Schwartz, G. E. Self-regulation of response patterning: Implications for psychophysiological research and therapy. *Biofeedback and Self-Regulation,* 1976, *1,* 7-30.

Smith, K. U., & Henry. J. P. Cybernetic foundations for rehabilitation. *American Journal of Physical Medicine,* 1967, *46,* 379-467.

Smith, K. U., & Smith, M. F. *Psychology: An introduction to behavior science.* Boston: Little, Brown & Co., 1973.

Tatton, W. G., & Lee, R. G. Evidence for abnormal long-loop reflexes in rigid Parkinsonian patients. *Brain Research,* 1975, *100,* 671-676.

Thorndike, E. L. Animal intelligence: An experimental study of the associative process in animals. *Psychological Monographs,* 1898, *2* (No. 8), 241, 242, 248. (In K. U. Smith & M. F. Smith *Psychology.* Boston: Little, Brown & Co., 1973).

ACKNOWLEDGMENTS

This research was supported by NINCDS Program Grant NS13974 and United Cerebral Palsy Grant R33-78.

9

Efficacy of Modified Palatal Lifts for Improving Resonance

James L. Aten
Alonzo McDonald
Marianne Simpson
Ray Gutierrez

INTRODUCTION

The literature contains numerous reports on the efficacy of utilizing palatal lifts for improving velopharyngeal competence since Gibbons and Bloomer (1958) introduced the procedure 25 years ago. Approximately 1 decade later, Hardy, Netsell, Schweiger, and Morris (1969) described speech gains in a cerebral palsied patient fitted with a lift, and Gonzalez and Aronson (1970) documented improvement in 35 patients with a variety of dysarthric conditions. Subsequent reports followed by Kipf-meuller and Lang (1972), who described changes in speech intelligibility and measured reduction in the size of velopharyngel lumen by radiographic cephalometric analysis, and by Kerman, Singer, and Davidoff (1973), in which they thoroughly assessed increased air flow rates and vital capacity changes in two patients. The consensus of the reviews supported the concept that palatal lift prostheses benefitted patients with velopharyngeal incompetence, particularly those with flaccid paralysis or paresis.

Gonzalez and Aronson (1970) cited limitations of a lift such as inadequate retention or intolerance of elevation when the soft palate is "very spastic or stiff." Clinicians have noted that the fixed, inflexible acrylic used to build the velar extension portion of the lift creates pressure from the cantilever effect of the velar tissue pressing on the posterior end of the lift. This pressure often necessitates retention clasps on the teeth to retain the prosthesis with resulting constant and possible excess pressure on the velum and dentition. The discomfort requires careful, gradual, and tedious additions of acrylic to the lift portion and may explain why some patients reject the lift before velopharyngeal closure is achieved, because of tissue irritation. These problems, plus the added weight from the extensive use of acrylic, render less than satisfactory results in the edentulous patient (Rosenbek & LaPointe, 1978), despite an earlier report (Lawshe, Hardy, Schweiger, & Van Allen, 1971) of successful lift retention in one edentulous patient.

The purpose of the present investigation was to evaluate the efficacy of specially designed palatal lifts in treating patients with a wide variety of neurological conditions resulting in major symptoms of hypernasal resonance, nasal emission, and severely impaired intelligibility. The traditional lift was modified so that the lift portion was attached to the body of a maxillary retainer or to existing dentures with wire connectors instead of the traditional solid acrylic. It was hypothesized that retention of such a modified lift would be enhanced.

SUBJECTS

Sixteen male patients, nine with dentures with a mean age of 55.4 years (range 40 to 69 years), served as subjects. All patients had moderate to severe dysarthria, a major component of which was hypernasal resonance. Table 9-1 shows ages, dental status, and etiologies. The majority of patients had incurred bilateral CVAs, resulting in varying dysarthria severities. Not all of the dysarthric speech samples were classifiable; however, the most common type was spastic dysarthria (Darley, Aronson, & Brown, 1975) as seen in Table 9-2. The majority of the 16 patients had demonstrable disturbances of articulation, respiration, and phonation that severely compromised intelligibility in conjunction with the abnormal nasal resonance.

PROCEDURAL OVERVIEW

The typical procedure for each patient began with an initial evaluation by a speech pathologist who determined that the patient's dysarthric symptomatology included excess nasal resonance as a major

TABLE 9-1.
Age, Dental Status, and Etiology for Dysarthric Patients. UMN = Upper Motor Neurone, LMN = Lower Motor Neurone.

Patient	Age	Dental Status	Etiology
1	57	Dentures	Bilateral CVA
2	61	Dentures	Bilateral CVA
3	56	Dentures	Ocular Muscular Dystrophy
4	54		ALS (Mixed UMN with Primarily LMN Component)
5	62	Dentures	Bilateral CVA
6	40		Collagen Disease, Ataxia
7	69	Dentures	Bilateral CVA
8	49		ALS (Mixed UMN & LMN)
9	55		Bilateral CVA
10	40	Dentures	Bilateral CVA
11	59		L CVA and Brain Stem Infarct
12	59		Bilateral CVA
13	63	Dentures	Bilateral CVA
14	45	Dentures	IX, X, XII Cranial Nerve Trauma (Gunshot Wound)
15	64		Bilateral CVA
16	53	Dentures	Bilateral CVA

component and that the patient's overall symptomatology made a clinical trial with a palatal lift appropriate. If a patient with appropriate symptoms volunteered to be a candidate for a palatal lift, referral was made to a prosthodonist who fabricated a lift attached by wires to either a maxillary retainer or the patient's denture. Next, clinical judgments of reduced nasal resonance/emission were made by a speech pathologist, and appropriate adjustments were performed to attain the best closure possible. Cineradiographic evaluations of velopharyngeal function, with and without the lift, were conducted and final adjustments were accomplished. Audio tape recordings, with and without the lift, were then made for subsequent judging. Some patients required a second visit to the prosthodontist to have acrylic added or, as was more often the case, to merely have the wire loops manipulated, followed by a second cineradiographic check on the actual lift position relative to maximal closure. The details of each procedure are specified below.

TABLE 9-2.
Dysarthria Classification (after Darley, Aronson, & Brown, 1975).

Patient	Classification
1	spastic dysarthria
2	spastic dysarthria and aphasia
3	flaccid dysarthria
4	mixed dysarthria (spastic, flaccid)
5	unclassified (?spastic dysarthria)
6	ataxic dysarthria (? mixed)
7	spastic dysarthria
8	mixed dysarthria
9	spastic dysarthria
10	spastic dysarthria
11	spastic dysarthria
12	spastic dysarthria
13	spastic dysarthria
14	flaccid dysarthria
15	spastic dysarthria
16	spastic dysarthria

Prosthetic Procedures

Each patient was referred to the prosthodontist who constructed the prosthesis. When natural teeth were present, a removable partial denture was designed to utilize existing teeth for retention of the palatal lift prosthesis. In patients who were edentulous, a complete denture was constructed with the acrylic lift connected by wires to the posterior border of the denture. The palatal lift portion was attached to the denture by two 18-gauge stainless steel, round wires with adjustment loops (See Figure 9-1). Adjustments could be made by the traditional addition or removal of acrylic from the lift or by adjusting the loops in the wire.

Cineradiographic Procedures

Each patient was evaluated cineradiographically after initial construction of the palatal lift to determine final adjustments of the anterior-posterior and superior dimensions of the lift to provide for the best preliminary closure possible based on visual inspections of velopharyngeal lumen size during speaking, sustained vowel phonations,

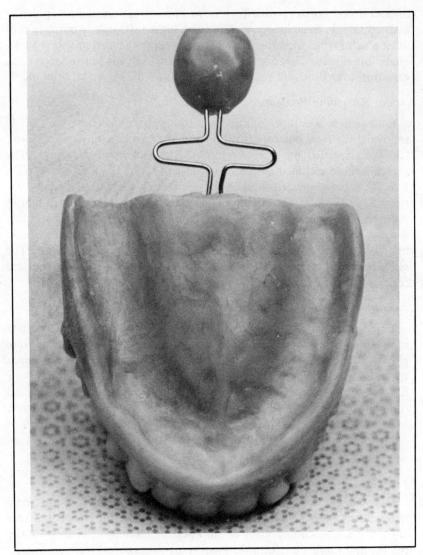

FIGURE 9-1
Palatal lift attached to dentures.

and swallowing. Additional evaluations consisted of perceptual judgments to ascertain significant reductions in hypernasal resonance and nasal emission. Foil was used to wrap the velar acrylic portion to increase visibility of the lift in contrast to tissue. Those patients who required gradual closure of the velopharyngeal lumen or who could not tolerate excess pressure initially, returned for a final cineradiographically assisted fitting. Sustained viewing of the spastic dysarthric patients producing contextual speech was necessary because they often showed adequate initial velar elevation on vowels or single words but reduced velar elevation over time and reduced velar motility during serial utterances.

Audio Recording Procedure

Each patient was tape recorded in a sound-isolated room immediately following the final palatal lift fitting and after a "best-possible closure" had been verified by cineradiography and perceptual judgment. The speech sample included sustained vowels (/a/, /i/, /u/); counting from 1 to 30; repeating words and sentences selected to sample plosives, affricates, and continuant/fricative consonants; and oral reading of a brief passage. Two speech samples were obtained, one with the lift and one without the lift. The audio tapes were edited and reproduced to obtain brief samples of counting and sentence production for later judging. The samples were randomized (with and without lift) for each patient and coded to prevent identification by the judges.

Judging Procedure

Three experienced speech pathologists served as judges. Tape recorded samples of patients counting and imitatively speaking sentences were played in a quiet, free-field environment, with each judge equidistant from the speaker. The judges were asked to decide whether sample A or B was perceived as changed on the dimension of reduced hypernasal resonance and to rate the degree of change, on a scale of *No Change, Mild Reduction, Moderate Reduction, Marked Reduction*. Judgments of relative amounts of nasal emission and of intelligibility were made on subsequent replays.

Vowel Duration Measures

Each sustained vowel was measured using a stop-watch (an admittedly quasiaccurate procedure) to estimate onset and cessation of voicing. This allowed relative comparisons of duration of phonation possible under the lift and nonlift conditions to assess air-wastage indirectly.

RESULTS

Hypernasal Resonance Changes

Counting. Of the 15[1] patients judged for hypernasal resonance, the judges unanimously agreed that 10 patients (66.7%) were improved while counting with the lift in place. A *moderate reduction* in hypernasality was judged for eight of these patients and a *mild reduction* for two. Four other patients were judged improved by two of the three judges. Two of these patients were judged as demonstrating a *mild reduction* and two a *moderate reduction.* Only one patient (P6) was judged to be more hypernasal while wearing the lift by two of the three judges. In summary, 14 of the 15 patients (93.3%) were judged by at least two raters to show mild to moderate reductions in hypernasal resonance while counting with the aid of the lift.

Sentence production. Eleven of the 16 patients (68.7%) were judged as less nasal in imitatively producing sentences with the lift. Five of these patients received ratings of *mild reduction,* and six patients were rated as showing *moderate reductions* in hypernasal resonance. Three other patients were judged as showing *mild reductions* in hypernasal resonance by two of the three judges, while one patient (P2) was judged to have *mild reduction* with the lift by one judge, no change by a second judge, and *mild reduction* without the lift by a third judge. Once again, (P6) was judged as speaking with more hypernasality when wearing the lift. In summary, 14 of the 16 patients (87.5%) were rated by at least two judges to show mild to moderate reductions in hypernasal resonance on sentence production with the lift in place.

The judges, in rating hypernasal resonance for counting and sentence production, demonstrated complete agreement on 71% of the samples. Complete disagreement between judges occurred in only one sample of the 93 possible.

Intelligibility of Sentences

Thirteen patients were evaluated by the three judges for intelligibility of speech while imitatively producing sentences. One-hundred percentage agreement was noted for only four patients. Three of these four patients were judged more intelligible with the lifts, while one patient was heard as more intelligible without the lift. Seven patients received two out of three ratings that were consistent, but only five of these were judged as more intelligibile with the lifts in place. Three patients received complete disparity of judgment (i.e., no difference, improved with the lift, improved without the lift). All of these patients had other problems that severely compromised articulatory production. In summary, the judges reported great difficulty in agreeing on the sample that was more intelligible, and this is supported by the objective findings of less than 30% total agreement among the judges. Obviously, the reduction of hypernasal resonance did not result in universal improvement in intelligibility. The patients for whom there was unanimous agreement frequently represented less severe involvement of other systems.

Nasal Emission

The greatest disparities in judging occurred in rating nasal emission, with reliability in this study being less than 20%. Seven patients (50%) were judged to have reduced nasal emission among the 14 rated with the lift. Four were rated as *no change,* and three were judged as having more nasal emission with the lift. Interjudge reliability was quite poor, with unanimous agreement in only two samples. Most judges stated that they could not discriminate nasal emission from other perceived variables such as breathiness, strain–strangled, or harsh voice quality.

Duration of Vowel Phonation

Duration measures for the three sustained vowels were numerically similar in estimating phonation time with and without lifts. Consequently, these were averaged for each of the two conditions. Patients averaged 5.7 sec of sustained vowel production without the lifts and 8.2 sec with the lifts. Only two patients had shorter vowel durations without lifts; these were patients with severe spastic dysarthria. Correlations between rated degree of intelligibility and increases in phonation time with lifts were small and statistically insignificant for the group. The variation among patients was high, ranging from 15.0 sec difference (patient with a major component of flaccid dysarthria) to .10 sec.

DISCUSSION

The palatal lifts were demonstrated to be effective in reducing hypernasal resonance for all but one of the patients as indicated by the judges' ratings. This was supported by our clinical impressions. The one patient (P6) judged consistently to be more hypernasal when wearing the lift was the patient subjectively perceived to have received no benefit from the appliance overall, including less vowel duration with the lift. He suffered from collagen disease and cerebellar dysfunction with ataxic speech and considerable variation in dysarthric symptomatology.

These results are compatible with Gonzalez and Aronson's report (1970) and others (Kipfmueller & Lang, 1972; Kerman et al., 1973) in showing the efficacy of palatal lifts. The results offer additional support for a conservative approach to ameliorating dysarthric speech symptoms as recommended by Darley et al. (1975) and Rosenbek and LaPointe (1978), particularly in patients who are high-risk surgical candidates.

The results for reduction of nasal emission were equivocal in this group of patients. The reason could have been that the judges needed listening training to isolate and discriminate this dimension. They expressed concerns such as, "I didn't know what to listen for!" It is undoubtedly difficult to recognize nasal emission in the presence of breathiness; reduced phonatory signals; harsh, strained vocal quality; and minimal articulatory movements. A related explanation appears equally plausible — namely, that nasal emission is better judged by instrumental (acoustic) measures rather than by perceptual measures (Fletcher, Sooudi, & Frost, 1974).

Changes in intelligibility were also hard to rate. Unanimous results were obtained for only four patients. Another five patients were judged more intelligible by two of the three judges for a total of 9 out of 13 patients. The most obvious reason for lack of improvement in three of the patients could be attributed to severe impairments of articulatory motility that compromised intelligible speech even when hypernasal resonance and/or nasal emission was reduced. Additionally, the patients who continued to receive treatment after lift fitting were not subsequently rated. Some of the patients in our group did continue to show clinical improvement in all dimensions of their dysarthric symptomatology.

The finding that phonation time on sustained vowels increased an average of 2 sec with the lift requires qualification.The patients with flaccid dysarthria (Ps 3, 4, 14) contributed the greatest to the group mean change. The patients with spastic dysarthria showed minimal change in phonation time with the lift, because of their inability to maintain respiratory flow and their increased vocal fold activity — often resulting in muteness after 2 to 3 sec of phonation. These spastic dysarthric patients were unable to produce sustained discourse or counting. Certain portions of their speech samples were inaudible and one patient reported increased tension throughout the speech tract with continued wearing of the lift — a report for which we clinically noted confirming evidence as phonation became inaudible.

In conclusion, the majority of the 16 patients had reductions in hypernasal resonance when wearing the lift. Some patients could communicate with their families and the medical center staff for the first time since the onset of their dysarthria. The degree of benefit varied considerably and seemed largely dependent upon the severity of involvement of other speech systems (i.e., respiratory, phonatory, articulatory). Follow-up visits indicated that initial tolerance of the lift was enhanced by gradually (over several days) elevating the lift and moving it in a posterior direction. Patients with active gag reflexes appeared to accommodate more readily to the lift. Irritated tissue was not a problem. Adjustments in the superior and posterior directions were simplified by manipulating the looped-wire connectors, rather than by adding acrylic as in the traditional, solid-acrylic palatal lift prosthesis. Denture seals were maintained and retention was not a major problem for our patients, unlike those reported by Rosenbek and LaPointe (1978). The results support the recommendations of Lawshe et al. (1971) for fitting patients who are edentulous and extend that recommendation to patients with other than flaccid velums. Some patients were able to eat with the lift in place. For those who were not able to eat with the lift, a second maxillary denture was fabricated without the lift portion of the prosthesis. Increased velar movement was noted in several patients after extended periods of wearing the lift. One patient with severe spastic dysarthria (P11) chose not to wear his lift after a lengthy trial period, because it increased the level of tonicity in laryngeal and pharyngeal musculature. The lift did have more immediate and persisting benefit for the patients with flaccid velums as noted by others; however, lifts can also offer some improvement for patients with other types of neurological impairment.

SUMMARY

Sixteen patients with heterogeneous dysarthric etiologies and symptomatologies were each fitted with palatal lifts. Nine of the patients were edentulous. The lift portion of the appliance consisted of acrylic attached to either the maxillary removable partial denture or complete denture by adjustable, loop-wire connectors. This permitted easy posterior and superior adjustments. Accommodation of the lift was no problem even for spastic dysarthric patients and retention of the maxillary denture was achieved in all nine edentulous patients. The majority of patients received benefit from the lift based on judged reduction of hypernasal resonance, improved intelligibility, and slightly increased phonation time. The modified lift, utilizing wire connectors is more easily adapted to dentures than the traditional solid acrylic palatal lift prosthesis. It may facilitate velar movements but that is to be determined by subsequent study.

NOTE

———————

[1]Sample sizes varied because not all patients produced audible samples on all tasks.

ACKNOWLEDGMENTS

We thank the Long Beach VA Medical Center for resources provided in support of this project. Thanks also to Dr. Emma Allen, Mrs. Sandra Davison-Baxter, and Dr. Jon Lyon for serving as judges (with great patience and perseverance) and to Dr. Wayne Thompson for his editorial assistance.

REFERENCES

Darley, F., Aronson, A., & Brown, J. *Motor speech disorders.* Philadelphia: Saunders, 1975.

Fletcher, S. Sooudi, I., & Frost, S. Quantitative and graphic analysis of prosthetic treatment for "nasalance" in speech. *Journal of Prosthetic Dentistry,* 1974, *32,* 284–291.

Gibbons, P., & Bloomer, H. A supportive-type prosthetic speech aid. *Journal of Prosthetic Dentistry,* 1958, *8,* 362–369.

Gonzalez, J., & Aronson, A. Palatal lift prosthesis for treatment of anatomic and neurologic palatopharyngeal insufficiency. *Cleft Palate Journal,* 1970, *7,* 91–104.

Hardy, J., Netsell, R., Schweiger, J., & Morris, H. Management of velopharyngeal dysfunction in cerebral palsy. *Journal of Speech and Hearing Disorders,* 1969, *34,* 123–137.

Kerman, P., Singer, L., & Davidoff, A. Palatal lift and speech therapy for velopharyngeal incompetence. *Archives of Physical Medicine Rehabilitation,* 1973, *54,* 271–276.

Kipfmueller, L., & Lang, B. Treating velopharyneal inadequacies with a palatal lift prosthesis. *Journal of Prosthetic Dentistry,* 1972, *27,* 63–72.

Lawshe, B., Hardy, J., Schweiger, J., & Van Allen, M. Management of a patient with velopharyngeal incompetency of undetermined origin: A clinical report. *Journal of Speech and Hearing Disorders,* 1971, *36,* 547–551.

Rosenbek, J., & LaPointe, L. The dysarthrias: Description, diagnosis, and treatment. In D. F. Johns (Ed.), *Clinical management of neurogenic communicative disorders.* Boston: Little, Brown, 1978.

Author Index

Subject Index